ASD

&

Me

ASD & Me

Publisher Jerry Coffey

© Jerry Coffey

All Rights Reserved

Table of Contents

Introduction : A personal Exploration of ASD: The inspiration Behind this Book

Chapter 1: Navigating Prosopagnosia: Living with Face Blindness

Chapter 2: Growing up with ASD: Reflections on How Autism Affected My Childhood

Chapter 3: Unpacking the AQ Test: Understanding the Autism Quotient Assessment

Chapter 4: Tracing the Genetics of ASD: Uncovering the Roots of Autism Spectrum Disorder

Chapter 5: Coping with ASD: Exploring Self-Medicating Strategies for Autism

Chapter 6: The Unique Abilities of Autistic Savants: An Insider's Perspective

Chapter 7: Accessing Support: Navigating Insurance Coverage for ASD Treatment

Chapter 8: ASD and the World of Music, Video Games, and Sports: Finding a Place to Thrive

Chapter 9: Finding Help: Organizations and Resources for Individuals with ASD

Chapter 10: My Journey to Diagnosis: Personal Reflections on Clinical Examinations for ASD

Chapter 11: Understanding Psychological Testing: A Guide to Different Types of Assessments

Chapter 12: Diagnosis Demystified: The Process of Standard Diagnostic Testing for ASD

Chapter 13: Love and Understanding: Navigating Relationships with an ASD Partner or Loved One

Introduction : A personal Exploration of ASD: The inspiration Behind this Book

ASD & Me is a personal and scientific exploration of Autism Spectrum Disorder. In this book, I offer a unique perspective as someone who has lived with ASD for my entire life. It will be of interest to anyone who has a personal connection to someone with ASD or suspects that they may have it themselves.

As I am now in my seventies, I reflect on how ASD has affected my life, and offer hope to parents of children with ASD that things can improve as coping mechanisms are developed. I offer myself as a specimen for this study due to the availability of a detailed medical record of brain imaging and diagnostic tests conducted throughout my life.

To provide a scientific analysis, I include written assessments from clinical psychologists, neurologists, neurosurgeons, and behavioral psychologists. I explain the tests they administered and provide a deep dive analysis of what they are meant to discover.

This book offers a unique and honest perspective on living with ASD and will be a valuable resource for those looking to understand and cope with the disorder.

In this book, we will delve into the technical aspects of genetic testing, including how it works and what it reveals.

I possess an inexplicable ability to learn difficult material quickly, as evidenced by my academic records. I offer these records as evidence that I am capable of functioning at a high level despite living with ASD, which I believe I have. While I have never received a formal diagnosis of ASD, I took the official autism test and scored 42 out of 50, with a score above 32 indicating the presence of ASD.

We will explore the various pharmaceutical solutions available for ASD patients, including the four main classes of drugs. In addition, we will cover common diagnostic examination procedures, such as reflex and memory tests. I sought to understand what the neurologist was looking for and what he discovered about my condition.

Overall, this book offers a comprehensive and honest examination of living with ASD, including its genetic and pharmaceutical aspects, diagnostic procedures, and personal experiences. It will be a valuable resource for those seeking to understand ASD and those affected by it.

Usually, a normal person would not publish their confidential medical reports particularly if they indicated Autism Spectrum Disorder.

My purpose in assembling these medical records is to look back and see if there were characteristic signs of ASD that were commented on but not recognized as ASD because ASD had not yet been defined.

I will include personal anecdotes that must have affected me greatly as I can still vividly recall the incidents. They are meant to illustrate situations that I found myself in because of my lack of ability in reading social cues and facial identity and expressions.

Perhaps this otherwise tedious study will be of interest to someone who wonders about the future of their son or daughter when they will be in their fifties and sixties.

Maybe some other seventy-year-old will read this and look back and see similarities in some of my confounding behaviors that seem to belie my intelligence.

The first time that I heard about Aspergers syndrome was when I was loading a tanker railcar with Bakken crude oil in North Dakota and passing the time talking with a railway worker. He told me about his sister with Asperger's and asked if I had ever heard about it. I wonder if he saw it in me and was talking about it because of how I acted. Anyway, that was when I first heard of ASD it was around 2010 or 2011. This is the first time in my life that I can take the time to do a deep dive into my head, brain, mind, personality, and actions.

Chapter 1: Navigating Prosopagnosia: Living with Face Blindness

For me, one of the most frustrating characteristics of my ASD is my inability to recognize faces. This has often led to awkward situations where I have failed to recognize people. The process of recognizing faces is a complex cognitive task that involves several regions of the brain. In my case, it seems that my Fusiform Gyrus, also known as the Fusiform Face Area (FFA), may not be functioning optimally. The FFA is a small area located in the lower part of the brain's temporal lobe, which is situated on the sides of the brain, just above the ears.

Due to the challenges, I face in recognizing faces, I have developed a range of coping mechanisms, such as paying attention to distinctive features like hairstyle, voice, and glasses. However, I still struggle with this aspect of my ASD, and it has impacted my social interactions throughout my life.

The FFA is a small, highly specialized area of the brain that is primarily involved in the recognition of faces and other complex visual stimuli. It is responsible for encoding the physical features of faces, including their shape, size, and orientation, as well as processing the emotional expressions conveyed by faces.

The FFA receives input from several other brain regions, including the primary visual cortex, the superior temporal sulcus, and the amygdala, which is involved in the processing of emotions. The superior temporal sulcus (STS) is a region of the brain located in the temporal lobe, specifically in the superior portion of the lateral sulcus. The superior portion of the lateral sulcus refers to a specific area in the brain, located in the temporal lobe, which is the part of the brain that's responsible for hearing, memory, and processing sensory information.

The lateral sulcus, also known as the Sylvian fissure, is a prominent groove that runs along the side of the brain, separating the temporal lobe from the frontal and parietal lobes. The superior portion of this groove is located toward the top of the temporal lobe and is called the superior temporal sulcus. This region is involved in many complex cognitive processes related to social cognition, such as perception and processing of social cues like facial expressions, body language, and voice intonation. It also plays a role in the perception of speech and language, particularly in the perception of prosody and the discrimination of phonetic sounds.

The STS has been shown to play a role in the perception of biological motion, gaze processing, and understanding the intentions of others. The STS is also implicated in the processing of speech and language, particularly in the perception of prosody and the discrimination of phonetic sounds. Prosody is a term used to describe the various patterns of rhythm, intonation, and emphasis in speech that contribute to conveying meaning beyond the words themselves. Essentially, it refers to how speech sounds, rather than just what it means. Prosody is a vital part of communication as it provides contextual information and indicates the speaker's emotions, attitudes, and intentions.

One important aspect of prosody is rhythm. Rhythm in speech is the pattern of stressed and unstressed syllables, which can differ depending on the language and dialect used. For example, in English, the word "banana" has the stress on the second syllable, while in Spanish, the stress is on the third syllable. Rhythm helps to make speech more musical and can contribute to making the language more engaging to listen to.

My lack of rhythm has been a constant in my life for as long as I can remember. When I was younger, I would try to dance along to my favorite songs, but my movements always felt stiff and awkward. Even something as simple as clapping along to the beat of a song felt impossible. As I got older, I tried to compensate for my lack of rhythm by learning to play musical instruments, first the piano and then the guitar. While I found the idea of reading sheet music fascinating, playing the instruments themselves was a challenge. No matter how much I practiced, my fingers never seemed to hit the right notes at the right time.

Both my mother and father were sergeants in the Army and Air Force, respectively, and they instilled a sense of discipline and order in our household. My brother, uncle, and cousin were also members of the Canadian Armed Forces. Although I admired their commitment to service and dedication to the country, I knew deep down that I could never follow in their footsteps. The idea of going through boot camp and participating in group marches filled me with dread. I knew that my lack of coordination and rhythm would make me a liability, and I would be the subject of ridicule among my peers. It was a painful realization, but one that I had to accept.

In a way, my struggles with rhythm and coordination have defined much of my life. It's an aspect of myself that I've had to come to terms with, and it's something that has both challenged and motivated me. It's given me a unique perspective on the world, and it's led me to pursue interests that don't rely on rhythm or coordination, like writing and photography.

Another aspect of prosody is intonation, which refers to the rising and falling of the pitch of the voice when speaking. Intonation can convey many different things, such as the difference between a statement and a question, or between a statement and a sarcastic remark. For example, a simple question like "Are you coming?" can be interpreted in many ways depending on the tone of voice used. A rising intonation at the end can indicate a genuine question, while a falling intonation can indicate surprise or disbelief.

Finally, emphasis is another important aspect of prosody. Emphasis is the way that we stress certain words or syllables to give them more importance in a sentence. This can be done in a variety of ways, such as by changing the pitch or volume of the voice. For example, in the sentence "I didn't say he stole my money," the emphasis can be changed to highlight different words and convey different meanings. By emphasizing "I," it indicates that someone else said it, not the speaker. By emphasizing "stole," it indicates that someone did take the money, just not necessarily the person being accused. By emphasizing "my," it indicates that it was the speaker's money that was taken, not someone else's.

Overall, prosody plays a crucial role in communication by allowing speakers to convey not only the meaning of their words but also their emotions, attitudes, and intentions. By using rhythm, intonation, and emphasis, speakers can convey different nuances of meaning and make their speech more engaging and effective.

Additionally, the STS is involved in the processing of emotional information and is implicated in the perception of emotions in others. Dysfunction of the STS has been linked to various neuropsychiatric conditions, such as autism spectrum disorders and schizophrenia, which are characterized by deficits in social cognition.

Studies using functional magnetic resonance imaging (fMRI) have shown that the FFA becomes more active when individuals are presented with faces than with other types of stimuli. Additionally, research has shown that damage to the FFA, either due to injury or disease, can result in a condition called prosopagnosia, which is the inability to recognize faces.

The FFA encodes the physical features of faces and processes emotional expressions conveyed by faces, while also receiving input from other brain regions involved in the processing of visual stimuli and emotions

One of the difficulties faced by individuals with prosopagnosia is recognizing friends and family members. They may not be able to recognize even those they are close to and may have to rely on other cues such as voice or clothing to identify people. This can lead to confusion and awkwardness in social situations, particularly if they do not know how to approach or interact with people they cannot recognize.

Another challenge for individuals with prosopagnosia is reading and understanding the emotions that others are expressing through their facial expressions. This can lead to misunderstandings in social situations and difficulty in interpreting the intentions and feelings of others. They may miss out on important emotional cues, which can lead to confusion and difficulty in building relationships with others.

Navigating social situations can also be difficult for people with prosopagnosia. For example, they may struggle in social situations such as parties or gatherings where they are expected to recognize and interact with people they may not have seen for a long time. This can lead to feelings of anxiety and social isolation, particularly if they are unable to recognize important people in their life.

In addition to these difficulties, individuals with prosopagnosia may struggle to remember people's names, even those they know well, due to difficulty in connecting names with faces. This can lead to embarrassment and frustration, particularly in social situations where they are expected to remember names and faces.

People with prosopagnosia may struggle with tasks that involve recognizing faces, such as remembering the faces of characters in a movie or identifying individuals in a crowd. This can limit their ability to enjoy certain activities and participate in everyday life.

It is important to note that prosopagnosia can vary in severity, and some individuals may experience only mild difficulties in recognizing faces, while others may have more significant impairments. There is currently no cure for prosopagnosia, but some people with the condition may find that strategies such as creating mental images or using memory aids can help them manage their difficulties.

Prosopagnosia, or face blindness, is a condition that affects many people, including some well-known public figures. Here are a few examples of famous people who have spoken publicly about their experience with prosopagnosia:

1. Brad Pitt: Brad Pitt has spoken openly about his difficulties recognizing faces and has said that he sometimes struggles to recognize even close friends and family members.
2. Jennifer Aniston: Jennifer Aniston has also spoken about her experience with prosopagnosia and has said that she often relies on other cues, such as voice or clothing, to recognize people.
3. Jane Goodall: The famous primatologist and conservationist Jane Goodall has also spoken about her experience with prosopagnosia. She has said that she has always struggled to recognize faces and that this has sometimes made social situations difficult for her.
4. Oliver Sacks: The late neuroscientist and writer Oliver Sacks wrote about his experience with prosopagnosia in his book "The Mind's Eye." Sacks described how his face blindness affected his personal and professional life, and how he learned to compensate for his difficulties.

5. Lisa Scottoline: Best-selling author Lisa Scottoline has also spoken publicly about her experience with prosopagnosia. She has said that her face blindness has sometimes made social situations difficult, but that she has learned to use other cues, such as voice or posture, to recognize people.

These are just a few examples of famous people who have spoken about their experience with prosopagnosia. While face blindness can be challenging, many people with the condition have learned to manage their difficulties and live full and successful lives.

Google Glasses, also known as Google Glass, are a wearable computer in the form of eyeglasses that were developed by Google. They feature a small, transparent display mounted on the side of the frame that can project images, videos, and information directly in front of the wearer's eyes. The glasses are controlled through a touchpad on the side of the frame, voice commands, or by using a smartphone app.

Google Glasses were designed to be a hands-free, augmented reality device that could provide users with real-time information, such as directions, weather, or even the ability to take photos or make video calls. Despite the initial hype surrounding the product, Google Glasses were discontinued in 2015 due to a lack of consumer interest and a number of concerns over privacy and safety.

There have been some studies that suggest that technology, such as Google Glasses, could potentially help people with face blindness. For example, a study conducted by researchers at the University of Oxford and the University of Cambridge found that participants with prosopagnosia were able to improve their ability to recognize faces using Google Glasses. In the study, participants were shown images of faces while wearing the glasses, and they were asked to identify the person in each image. The researchers found that participants who used Google Glasses performed significantly better than those who did not.

The study conducted by researchers at the University of Oxford and the University of Cambridge was published in the Journal of Medical Internet Research in 2016. The study involved a small group of participants with prosopagnosia, and it aimed to determine whether Google Glasses could be used to improve their ability to recognize faces. The study found that participants who used Google Glasses performed significantly better at recognizing faces than those who did not use the technology.

Another study conducted at Harvard Medical School found that participants with prosopagnosia who used Google Glasses were able to recognize faces more accurately than those who did not use the technology. The study involved training participants to use Google Glasses to recognize people, and the results showed that participants were able to improve their ability to recognize faces over time. The study conducted at Harvard Medical School was published in the Journal of Assistive Technologies in 2017.

The study involved a larger group of participants with prosopagnosia, and it aimed to investigate the potential benefits of using Google Glasses for individuals with the condition. The study found that participants who used Google Glasses were able to recognize faces more accurately than those who did not use the technology. Additionally, the study showed that participants who used the technology improved their ability to recognize faces over time as they became more familiar with the device.

These studies suggest that technology, such as Google Glasses, could be a useful tool for people with prosopagnosia. However, it is important to note that more research is needed to fully understand the potential benefits and limitations of this technology for individuals with face blindness. Additionally, it is important to consider the potential ethical and privacy concerns associated with using technology like Google Glasses to recognize faces.

Many times, I have not recognized someone that I should have, and they wondered why. They think I am snubbing them, or I am somehow rejecting them, but I simply do not recognize their faces.

An extreme example happened to me at one job when I was a trucker. I was introduced to my new dispatchers. Two females in their mid thirties. I noted things about them. Their glasses, coffee mugs, car keyrings, slippers, desk chairs, computer setups and so on.

Later I was talking alone to one dispatcher about how her husband had brought her some rare perogy flavoured potato chips and how she didn't want to open the one-of-a-kind package. Both dispatchers were very nice women but there was a peculiarity of sorts with one woman who had a bald head and a right eye that stared way too far up all of the time.

I left the room and when I returned unbeknownst to me the other dispatcher came into the room when the one, I had been talking to left. She saw the potato chip bag and ripped it open thinking nothing of it. I said how shocked I was that she changed her mind. She stood up and looked me in the face and correctly accused me of thinking that she was the other girl.

Chapter 2: Growing up with ASD: Reflections on How Autism Affected My Childhood

ASD has had a significant impact on every aspect of my life, but it does not define who I am. It wasn't until I was in my seventies that I realized I had been living with ASD for my entire life. Looking back, I can see that my challenges began in grade one when my teacher instructed my classmates to report me if I was seen 'daydreaming.' I felt this was unfair and worried that my mother would find out.

I remember a particular incident from grade one when all of us kids were lined up at the water fountain in the hallway. As we were walking into the classroom, I asked the teacher if she thought that I could shinny up a support column in the hallway. She sarcastically answered, "Why yes Jerry, we will all go into the classroom, and you can climb up the pole." Thinking that I was with the group, she closed the door leaving me alone in the hall by the pole.

I climbed up the pole and slid back down. When I realized that I was alone in the hallway I walked home. Little did I know at the time that the teacher's response was sarcastic and not a genuine encouragement. I took everything people said to be true. If my mother told me that a 'little bird' had told her what I had done I would totally believe her and wonder which one.

After the incident at school, I had to face another traumatic experience when our house burned down. It was a very close call for all of us, and it was an experience that has stayed with me to this day. I was just a six-year-old boy, and my mother was holding my baby brother Teddy when the fire started. In addition to my mother and baby brother my two younger sisters Maxine and Linda were all standing in the living room. A very heroic neighbour lady happened to be outside at the time, and she ran into the burning building to help my mother get us out. She told my mother to give her the baby and get the two little girls.

As the flames quickly spread up the walls of the living room, I felt a deep sense of fear that I had never experienced before. The smoke was thick and suffocating, it choked us, and it burned our eyes and filled our lungs. I remember feeling completely helpless as I struggled to find a way out. My mother was calling out to me "Jerry open the door. Open the door." But I couldn't see anything through the dense smoke. In the chaos of the moment, I got tangled up in the drapes and started to panic. It felt like an eternity, but we all eventually made it out unharmed.

We had to move into a trailer after that, and it was a difficult time for my family. But we were grateful to be alive and to have each other. That experience has stayed with me for my entire life, and it's a reminder to cherish every moment and to be grateful for what I have.

The six of us moved into a 7 by 35-foot trailer, and I needed to go to a new school. On my first day at the new school on Pembina highway in Winnipeg the kids started taunting me. Because my name is Coffey and I had bright red hair they were making reference to the well-known Maxwell House coffee advertisement about the coffee with the red star on top.

I acted badly when the most aggressive bully charged at me thinking he would knock me down to the ground. I placed both my hands on his head and smashed his face into the corner of the red brick school wall. His face was bloody, and he was wailing loudly; and all the kids that thought they were going to bully me for the rest of the school year fled into the school.

I ran all the way home because I thought that I was going to get in trouble. My mother asked why I was home early. I told her that kids at the school had tried to fight with me. She thought that I had run and that they had chased me. But from that day on I have never once ran from people who have wanted to hurt me. I never went back to that school again. I think I was expelled for a year.

Our family moved to Portage la Prairie about seventy miles west of Winnipeg. I got along very well there, and I have fond memories of my childhood in the small town and at the Southport air force base. School went well in Portage and two different schools treated me fairly with no incidents.

My father was transferred with the Royal Canadian Air Force to Baden-Soellingen Germany in 1957. Things did not go as well there.

When I started attending the large school building that housed grades K through 12, I was in fourth grade and already a bit overweight at ten or eleven years old. Back then, the ultimate symbol of cool was the James Dean-style rebel on a motorcycle, complete with black boots and a black leather jacket.

Determined to be cool, I saved up my hard-earned pin-setting wages from the base bowling alley and splurged on a pair of black, thick-soled, chrome-buckled Wellington boots. However, my fashion sense was quickly quashed when the teachers banned me from wearing them to school. They even went as far as to make announcements over the school PA system to all students, warning them not to wear Wellington boots to school.

We all lived right on a military base, and I successfully argued that Wellington boots were allowed as formal wear for officers. After presenting my case to the school principal, I was allowed to wear them to school, and many other boys followed suit.

One day, when our regular arithmetic teacher was absent, Mr. Metivier, a substitute teacher with a heavy French accent, took over the class. He wrote a simple math problem on the blackboard: 8 + 6 = ? Turning to me, he demanded an answer in a condescending and cross tone: "Coffey, what is the answer?" I replied confidently, "Fourteen."

Instead of acknowledging my correct response, Mr. Metivier launched into a tirade of insults aimed directly at me. He bellowed, "Fourteen what? Apples? Oranges?" and then proceeded to belittle me further, shouting "You lazy, lousy, fat slug." Mr. Metivier's unprovoked attack left me feeling embarrassed in front of my friends and classmates.

Despite Mr. Metivier's insults, I refused to let him get the better of me. In fact, it was the first time that I had ever stood up to an adult in my life. Rather than lash out in anger or respond to his insults, I simply turned my back on him and got up from my desk and walked slowly out the classroom door in silence.

As I made my way down the empty hallway, I heard the distinct sound of my Wellington boots echoing through the school. I resisted the urge to run or hurry my pace, instead letting my calm and deliberate footsteps announce my departure to anyone who might be listening.

I wasn't content to simply let the matter rest there. With the support of my parents, I lodged a complaint with the school authorities, and the school board ultimately made the surprising decision to appoint

Mr. Metivier as the new school principal that very week.

Mr. Metivier called me into his office soon after he settled in and closed the door. Behind the door was a large rack of brass hooks with door keys on every hook. There were dozens of hooks. Without saying a word, he grabbed me by the lapels with both hands and lifted me high off my feet and then rammed my back onto the peg board as hard as he could with a menacing look in his eyes.

I never told anyone about what he did until today as I am writing this. I did not want to get my dad kicked off of the air force base. We would have been immediately posted back to somewhere unknown in Canada. My whole family would have to move because of me.

The reason that I was so worried about my father's military career was because of something that had happened the previous week. My father came home from work at the base and he was absolutely livid. He told me that he had risked his life many times in World War II and that he has served in the RCAF for nearly ten years without incident. He said that he was months away from his ten-year medal that would probably help him obtain the rank of sergeant from the corporal that he was at the time.

He crossly related how he had been 'on the carpet' which is military speak for being called in for an interview with the base Warrant Officer. Now on his promotion evaluation it would be noted that he 'had been on the carpet'. I was the reason that the Warrant Officer had summonsed my father. I see it now as an early indication of my ASD.

My family attended the Protestant church on the military base every Sunday morning. There were two identical churches at either end of the long block with separate parking lots and walkways. Attendees of one church never ever saw parishioners of the other church and vice versa for the Catholics. It was something that no one ever talked about or even noticed.

So, one weekday I waited at the Catholic church until the priest came by and I asked to talk to him. I told him that part of my family were practicing Roman Catholics and part were Protestants. There was no family record of how my side left the Catholic church to become Protestants. The priest gave me a rosary and a Missal book about the church and I left feeling that my questions had been answered. But the priest must have reported me to the Warrant Officer as a potential troublemaker. No one else had ever questioned such things before.

Mr. Metivier had a teacher named Mr. Alexander bully me for him. They gave me an hour detention after school every day for the rest of the year although I did nothing wrong to deserve it.

In class Mr. Alexander would frequently sneak up behind me and hit me as hard as he could on my knuckles with a wooden steel-edged yardstick. I reached a serious breaking point. I was prepared for him to lean over me to get a good aim with his yardstick. Then I let him hit me but this time I pretended that a reflex reaction caused my elbow to jerk back and accidentally crush his Adam's apple. I missed by an inch but when he looked into my eyes, he saw that I intended to drop him right there on the spot. He never assaulted me again.

I had Mr. Proctor, a very fair principal at Victoria Composite High School in Edmonton, Alberta. One day he called me into his office, and he said to me. "You are the smartest student in this whole school. I am not going to be known as the principal that kicked someone with as high an IQ as you out of school. Ever."

My attendance was horrendous I missed more than 200 days per year for three years. I spent my time alone in downtown pool halls, reading the Daily Digest horse racing forms handicapping horseraces which I would later place bets on at the Northlands Park racetrack where I went every evening.

Spending hours with the daily racing forms which had the statistics for recent horseraces and statistics about trainer and jockey standings and prices for horses at claiming races was something that I love doing. Through the numbers I can visualize the races and pit horse against horse in imaginary matchups. My skills at handicapping got better and better and I read every book on the subject that I could find at the Edmonton libraries.

Besides trying to predict which horse would win I was able to calculate odds in my head as the tote board odds were constantly changing in the minutes leading up to the horserace and the various totals that were accruing in the pools for daily doubles, exacta betting, and quinellas. I would change my bet as the situation unfolded.

I could easily pass the high school exams without going to the classes and doing homework, but the teachers resented me so much they gave me poor grades. I complained to my mother. She came up with a plan. An older student Bruce Robinson who lived a few doors down had taken the English class two years earlier from the same elderly female teacher. Bruce had made two spelling errors and had been deducted two points for a final score of 77%. My mother had me write the exact same words that Bruce had turned in with no spelling errors. The teacher gave my paper a grade of 44%, a failing grade. In English no less in what should have been my best subject.

When we showed Mr. Proctor, he held a meeting with the teacher. He said I could quit her class or continue. I said that I wished to continue but that I hoped the grading would be done more fairly. She failed me for the year anyway.

I became upset and thought the system was rigged against me. I quit school and enrolled in Alberta correspondence courses. One term assignment was to produce a plan to revitalize a primitive Caribbean Island. You have to understand that at this time the only gambling other than at the racetrack was church basement bingos and the annual Irish Sweepstakes.

In my paper I suggested that the imaginary island could promote gambling as a source of revenue and could offer Swiss style secret bank accounts and become a tax haven. I think I may have mentioned the possibility of marketing cannabis tourism like Jamaica had a reputation for. The correspondence markers threatened to expel me if I ever said anything like that again. Today I look at the Caribbean and see exactly what I was suggesting way back then in 1965.

In any event I scored an 'A' on one correspondence course and an "A-" on the other. This was because for the first time I got a fair assessment of my work. This was the first time I ever had the satisfaction of scoring an 'A.'

When I asked the Alberta Department of Education to consolidate the correspondence course with the regular courses so that I could graduate they said the correspondence courses grades were too low to count, then they said the grades were lost. Then they said one was a 'D' and the other a 'C-' and that I would not receive any diploma.

So, I forgot about the high school diploma and went to the University of Winnipeg as an adult admit student without it. Earlier in 1973 I had obtained an

'A+' in Economics 101 and an 'A' in psychology 101 from the extension division of the University of Manitoba. I was allowed to transfer these grades towards my studies at the University of Winnipeg.

I graduated from the University of Winnipeg with a three-year Bachelor of Arts degree majoring in Administrative Studies in 1990. I had scored A's in several more full- credit courses, and several half-year courses and was designated with the 'Student of Distinction' accreditation on my transcripts.

In 2016 I received a few more full credit course 'A's at the University of British Columbia's Sauder School of Business where I took a two-year program to obtain my CRA certificate a Certified Residential Appraiser from the Appraisal Institute of Canada.

Later in 2018 I wanted to learn how to program computers, so I studied for two years at the University of Winnipeg Applied Computer Science Department until Covid hit. I managed to score a couple more 'A's along with a few repeated classes; but I learned how to do advanced computer coding and passed. This happened when I was in my late sixties and most of my fellow students were surprised as were the professors.

This information was not meant as a life-list made by a grievance collector, but as a demonstration of some of the problems that my ASD caused me before I even knew what it was or that I had it.

Chapter 3: Unpacking the AQ Test: Understanding the Autism Quotient Assessment

Asperger's syndrome was once considered a distinct condition under the autism spectrum disorder (ASD) umbrella. However, in 2013, Asperger's was officially reclassified as a high functioning form of autism by the American Psychiatric Association (APA) in the fifth edition of its Diagnostic and Statistical Manual of Mental Disorders (DSM-5).

Autism Spectrum Disorder (ASD) is a neurodevelopmental disorder characterized by difficulties in social communication, repetitive behaviors, and restricted interests. It affects 1 in 59 individuals in the United States. The autism spectrum is wide and diverse, encompassing individuals with varying levels of abilities and challenges.

The change from Asperger's to Autism Spectrum Disorder reflects a shift in understanding and diagnosing autism. Prior to the DSM-5, Asperger's was seen as a separate condition from autism, with individuals diagnosed with Asperger's often thought of as having milder symptoms compared to those diagnosed with autism. However, research has shown that there are no significant differences in terms of symptoms between individuals with Asperger's and those with autism, leading to the conclusion that Asperger's should be considered a subtype of autism.

The DSM-5 criteria for diagnosing autism spectrum disorder include two core domains: impairments in social communication and social interaction, and restricted, repetitive patterns of behavior, interests, or activities. The criteria also include the presence of symptoms in early childhood, although they may not be fully manifested until social demands exceed the individual's abilities.

The change from Asperger's to Autism Spectrum Disorder has resulted in a more accurate and comprehensive understanding of the condition, leading to better support and resources for individuals on the autism spectrum. It also promotes greater understanding and acceptance of the diverse range of individuals who experience autism and recognizes that autism is a spectrum with a wide range of symptoms, abilities, and challenges.

However, the change has also led to some concerns and challenges. Some individuals who were previously diagnosed with Asperger's may feel that they are losing their identity with the reclassification. Additionally, the DSM-5 criteria may result in some individuals being misdiagnosed or not receiving a diagnosis at all, particularly those with high functioning autism who may not meet the full criteria for the disorder.

Here are twenty common symptoms of Autism Spectrum Disorder (ASD) in adults:

1. Difficulty with social interactions and relationships

2. Avoidance of eye contact

3. Lack of understanding of social cues

4. Repetitive behaviours or routines

5. Fixation on specific interests

6. Difficulty with change or transitions

7. Verbal and nonverbal communication difficulties

8. Difficulty with expressing emotions

9. Poor perspective taking

10. Lack of empathy

11. Inability to understand sarcasm or humor

12. Difficulty with abstract concepts

13. Limited interests

14. Sensory sensitivities

15. Avoidance of physical touch

16. Inability to recognize personal boundaries

17. Self stimulating behaviour (rocking, nail biting)

18. Narrow or intense interests

19. Poor organization and time management

20. Difficulty making and keeping friends

This is the AQ test used by professionals for diagnosis.

I will give my honest thought processes for the test. Firstly, it is especially important for me to get 100% on the test as usual. I will try to get a 'read' on the creator of the test by analyzing the questions for bias and will be looking for trick questions.

I think in terms of true or not true. There is no slightly true, it is either true or not true to me, although I can understand slightly false.

1. I prefer to do things with others rather than on my own.

My Answer Definitely Disagree: of course

2. I prefer to do things the same way over and over again.

My Answer Definitely Agree: much safer and more efficient.

3. If I try to imagine something, I find it very easy to create a picture in my mind.

My Answer Definitely Disagree: I need it on paper to see it clearly like diagrams, notes, pictures.

4. I frequently get so strongly absorbed in one thing that I lose sight of other things.

My Answer Definitely Agree: that's normal

5. I often notice small sounds when others do not.

My Answer Definitely Agree: I don't tell the others.

6. I usually notice car number plates or similar strings of information

My Answer Definitely Agree: but I am not memorizing them.

7. Other people frequently tell me that what I've said is impolite, even though I think it is polite.

My Answer Definitely Agree: I blurt out controversial opinions and will say bad things about other people behind their backs or ask inappropriate questions.

8. When I'm reading a story, I can easily imagine what the characters might look like.

My Answer Definitely Disagree: I cannot imagine any faces even the faces of people that I know of like actors.

9. I am fascinated by dates.

My Answer Definitely Agree: Who isn't?

10. In a social group, I can easily keep track of several different people's conversations.

My Answer Definitely Agree: I try to eavesdrop.

11. I find social situations easy.

My Answer Slightly Agree: I can cope ok.

12. I tend to notice details that others do not.

My Answer Definitely Agree: They say that to me.

13. I would rather go to a library than to a party.

My Answer Definitely Agree: anywhere but a party.

14. I find making up stories easy.

My Answer Definitely Agree: I authored a 384-page novel.

15. I find myself drawn more strongly to people than to things.

My Answer Definitely Disagree: I am not drawn to things or people.

16. I tend to have very strong interests, which I get upset about if I can't pursue.

My Answer Definitely Agree

17. I enjoy social chitchat.

My Answer Definitely Disagree: I might blurt and all they are looking for is ammo to talk about me later.

18. When I talk, it isn't always easy for others to get a word in edgewise.

My Answer Slightly Agree: My wife accuses me of that.

19. I am fascinated by numbers.

My Answer Definitely Agree: Numbers I understand.

20. When I'm reading a story, I find it difficult to work out the characters' intentions.

My Answer Definitely Agree: I don't try to guess ahead what characters will do later in the story.

21. I don't particularly enjoy reading fiction.

My Answer Slightly Disagree: I have read hundreds of novels, but I prefer Biographies and non-fiction.

22. I find it hard to make new friends.

My Answer Definitely Agree: That is because I do not trust new people.

23. I notice patterns in things all the time.

My Answer Definitely Agree: I look for patterns.

24. I would rather go to the theater than to a museum.

My Answer Slightly Disagree: This is a tough one. If I go to a theater I go late so there are no crowds at the concessions and it is dark so I can anonymously find a seat away from anyone and can be reasonably assured no one will sit near me. I worry about cleanliness and bedbugs. As for a museum I prefer that because I can choose a slow day and find exhibits that are quiet and have few other guests.

25. It does not upset me if my daily routine is disturbed.

My Answer Definitely Disagree: Daylight savings time disturbs my rhythm for a week or more after.

26. I frequently find that I don't know how to keep a conversation going.

My Answer Definitely Agree: I think maybe I should stop talking and leave on a good note before I put my foot in my mouth.

27. I find it easy to "read between the lines" when someone is talking to me.

My Answer Definitely Disagree: I do not get inuendo. I take everything someone says literally.

28. I usually concentrate more on the whole picture, rather than on the small details.

My Answer Definitely Disagree: I focus on details first.

29. I am not very good at remembering phone numbers.

My Answer Definitely Agree:

30. I don't usually notice small changes in a situation or a person's appearance.

My Answer Definitely Disagree: Because I have such poor facial recognition I use purses, and glasses, hairstyles, and cars to help identify coworkers.

31. I know how to tell if someone listening to me is getting bored.

My Answer Definitely Disagree:

32. I find it easy to do more than one thing at once.

My Answer Definitely Disagree: If I am talking on the phone and someone around me talks to me, I forget who I am on the phone with and what we were saying.

33. When I talk on the phone, I'm not sure when it's my turn to speak.

My Answer Definitely Agree: But isn't that just cell phones?

34. I enjoy doing things spontaneously.

My Answer Definitely Disagree:

35. I am often the last to understand the point of a joke.

My Answer Definitely Agree: I hate jokes and I most often don't laugh even if I do get them.

36. I find it easy to work out what someone is thinking or feeling just by looking at their face.

My Answer Definitely Disagree: I get no cues from facial expressions at all. It is a real problem for me.

37. If there is an interruption, I can switch back to what I was doing very quickly.

My Answer Definitely Agree: I ignore the distraction.

38. I am good at social chitchat.

My Answer Definitely Disagree: Trick question?

39. People often tell me that I keep going on and on about the same thing.

My Answer Definitely Disagree: There are no people, but my wife does say that sometimes.

40. When I was young, I used to enjoy playing games involving pretending with other children.

My Answer Definitely Disagree: I cannot remember but I doubt it. We played capture the flag war games a lot.

41. I like to collect information about categories of things (e.g., types of cars, birds, trains, plants).

My Answer Definitely Agree: I have Sibley's, Stokes, Audubon , and the Peterson Field Guide bird books with a current lifelist.

42. I find it difficult to imagine what it would be like to be someone else.

My Answer Definitely Agree: Impossible to do.

43. I like to carefully plan any activities I participate in.

My Answer Definitely Agree:

44. I enjoy social occasions.

My Answer Definitely Disagree: But I can function ok and fit in. I do not like to be near alcohol drinking.

45. I find it difficult to work out people's intentions.

My Answer Definitely Agree: I never wonder about other people's thoughts or what they will do next.

46. New situations make me anxious.

My Answer Definitely Disagree: I don't care what happens.

47. I enjoy meeting new people.

My Answer Definitely Disagree: I have the face problem, my blurting, and eccentric opinions

48. I am a good diplomat.

My Answer Definitely Disagree:

49. I am not very good at remembering people's date of birth.

My Answer Definitely Agree:

50. I find it very easy to play games with children that involve pretending.

My Answer Definitely Disagree: I avoid children.

My score was 42 out of 50. Scores in the 33-50 range indicate significant Autistic traits. When I first took a similar test with similar results, I felt somewhat relieved that there was a condition to account for some of my peculiarities. I had always suspected that something was off.

In 1973 when I was twenty-two years old, I attended a two-week psychological assessment that will be described later in detail.

In 1997 when I was forty-five years old, I was assessed by The Department of Clinical Psychology at the University of Saskatchewan where Mirna Vrbancic Ph. D a registered psychologist conducted extensive testing on me to determine if I had a learning disability.

In 2004 when I was fifty-five years old, I suffered a TBI traumatic brain injury, and the Emergency Room at the Health Sciences Hospital in Winnipeg took a CT brain scan without infusion and an MRI scan of my head.

I was under the care of Dr. Stefan Pacin M.D. FRCPC Neurology a neurologist in Winnipeg and over two years I took many PET , EEG scans and behavioral tests.

In 2010 when I was sixty years old. I self-diagnosed an adenoma of my pituitary gland, and my neurosurgeon took three MRI scans.

I am in between two books that I am self publishing. *Bitcoin for the Boardroom* and *Diesel Diaries* which I am editing for Barbara Stevenson my lifelong companion. I have published three books now starting in 2018 with *Bitcoin Billionaire: Bitcoin and Blockchain Wealth Creation*.

I wrote my first novel *Fetchers of Water : The Panda Polar Bear War* in 2020. The first book was written about people as an observer might do, I patterned my writing after Ken Auletta from *Vanity Fair* whose 2010 book *Googled : The end of the world as we know it*. Which I enjoyed so much. I watched the many young people that I wrote about on YouTube and in person at conferences but did not attempt to meet or interview any of them.

For my novel I had to create believable characters and bring them to life with personalities relationships and families. In writing *Fetchers of Water,* I wrote in 'character arc' without knowing that it existed as a requirement of good writing. This is where the characters are personally changed by the situations, they go through that are detailed in the story.

My novel did not sell well, and I found quite a reluctance for people to read it. Today a 384-page book is out of range for most people. I thought it was well worth the year it took to write the novel and I am proud of it and what it says.

In accordance with the honesty factor in this book I will reveal something. I wrote in dozens of predictions into the plot of *Fetchers of Water* that were unknowable on the date that the book was published. For me, the most relevant prediction was that the Canada United States Border would be closed between Manitoba and North Dakota and Minnesota; but there are dozens more.

The book was billed as an Eco Thriller spy novel and in my opinion would be an interesting read for everyone. My insight into the looming water crisis could be a result of my thinking differently than most people who are oblivious and unconcerned about future water shortages in so many parts of the world.

Chapter 4: Tracing the Genetics of ASD: Uncovering the Roots of Autism Spectrum Disorder

Autism Spectrum Disorder is a complex neurodevelopmental disorder that has been the subject of extensive research over the past several decades. Studies have consistently indicated that there is a strong genetic component to the development of autism, although the exact causes of the disorder are still not fully understood.

One of the most compelling lines of evidence for a genetic component to autism is the high rate of concordance seen in twin studies. In these studies, if one identical twin is diagnosed with autism, there is a 90% likelihood that the other twin will also be diagnosed with the condition. This provides convincing evidence that genetic factors play a role in the development of autism.

Polymerase Chain Reaction (PCR) is an extremely sensitive molecular biology technique used to amplify specific segments of DNA. The technique was first described in 1985 by Kary Mullis and has since become an essential tool in genetic research, diagnostics, and forensics.

The principle of PCR is based on the use of a thermostable DNA polymerase enzyme, which can withstand the high temperatures required for denaturation and annealing of DNA. The polymerase enzyme is combined with a DNA template, primers, nucleotides, and buffer in a thermal cycler machine. The thermal cycler machine allows for precise control of temperature and time, which are critical for the PCR reaction.

The PCR reaction consists of three steps: denaturation, annealing, and extension. During denaturation, the double-stranded DNA template is heated to a high temperature (usually 94-98°C), which causes the two strands to separate, resulting in single-stranded DNA. In the annealing step, the temperature is lowered to allow the primers to bind to their complementary sequences on the template DNA.

The primers are short DNA sequences that define the start and end of the region to be amplified. During the extension step, the temperature is raised to allow the DNA polymerase enzyme to synthesize a complementary strand to the template DNA using the primers as a starting point. This step produces a double-stranded DNA molecule that contains the region of interest.

After one cycle of denaturation, annealing, and extension, the PCR reaction has doubled the amount of DNA in the sample. The PCR process is then repeated for many cycles (usually 20-40 cycles) to exponentially amplify the region of interest. Each cycle of PCR produces a new copy of the DNA molecule, resulting in a large number of copies of the specific DNA segment.

PCR has many applications in molecular biology, including DNA sequencing, gene expression analysis, and the detection of genetic mutations. PCR can also be used in clinical diagnostics to detect the presence of infectious agents, such as bacteria and viruses, and to detect genetic abnormalities, such as chromosomal translocations and deletions. The development of real-time PCR, which allows for the monitoring of the PCR reaction in real-time, has further expanded the use of PCR in diagnostic testing.

The CRISPR DNA sequencing machine is a recent technology that uses the CRISPR/Cas system to accurately sequence DNA in a fast, efficient, and cost-effective manner. The CRISPR/Cas system is a naturally occurring mechanism found in bacterial cells that provides immunity against invading viruses by targeting and cutting viral DNA. This system has been adapted and repurposed to create a precise and reliable method for sequencing DNA.

The CRISPR DNA sequencing machine consists of three main components: a guide RNA (gRNA), a CRISPR-associated protein (Cas), and a fluorescent reporter molecule. The gRNA is designed to specifically target the region of interest in the DNA sequence to be analyzed. The Cas protein is then used to cut the DNA at specific locations determined by the gRNA. After the DNA is cut, the fluorescent reporter molecule is released and detected, allowing for the precise identification of the DNA sequence.

The CRISPR DNA sequencing machine operates in a cyclic process of targeting, cutting, and detecting. In each cycle, the gRNA is used to target the specific DNA sequence to be analyzed. The Cas protein then cuts the DNA at the target location, which releases the fluorescent reporter molecule. The amount of fluorescent reporter molecule released is proportional to the number of DNA molecules cut at the target location. This process is repeated multiple times, each time targeting a different part of the DNA sequence, until the entire sequence has been analyzed.

The CRISPR DNA sequencing machine has several advantages over traditional sequencing methods. It is more efficient and faster, as the CRISPR/Cas system can be programmed to target specific DNA sequences, eliminating the need for amplification of the DNA sample. This reduces the time required for sequencing and the potential for errors caused by amplification. Additionally, the CRISPR DNA sequencing machine is highly accurate, as the system can be programmed to target specific regions of the genome, reducing the potential for off-target effects and errors.

The CRISPR DNA sequencing machine has many applications in genetic research, diagnostics, and personalized medicine. It can be used to sequence the entire genome, identify specific genetic mutations, and detect infectious agents in clinical samples. The technology has the potential to revolutionize the field of genomics by enabling fast, efficient, and cost-effective sequencing of DNA.

Additionally, advances in genetic research have led to the identification of specific genetic variants that have been associated with an increased risk for autism. These include rare, high-impact mutations in specific genes, as well as common, low-impact variations in multiple genes that contribute to autism risk in a cumulative manner.

For example, mutations in the SHANK3 gene have been consistently linked to autism, while common variations in multiple genes have been associated with an increased risk for the disorder. SHANK3 is a gene that is located on chromosome 22 and encodes a protein of the same name. This protein is a scaffolding protein that is important for the formation and function of synapses in the brain. Synapses are the junctions between nerve cells that allow for communication and the transfer of information.

SHANK3 is particularly important for the proper functioning of the postsynaptic density.

Phelan-McDermid syndrome is characterized by neonatal hypotonia, absent to severely delayed speech, developmental delay, and minor dysmorphic facial features. Most affected individuals have moderate-to-profound intellectual disability. Other features include large fleshy hands, dysplastic toenails, and decreased perspiration that results in a tendency to overheat. Normal stature and normal head size distinguish Phelan-McDermid syndrome from other autosomal chromosome disorders. Behavior characteristics include mouthing or chewing non-food items, decreased perception of pain, and autism spectrum disorder or autistic-like affect and behavior.

HANK3 is a gene that is essential for the development and function of the brain. The gene provides instructions for making a protein called Shank3, which is critical for the communication between brain cells. The Shank3 protein is made up of different building blocks or exons, with 22 of these exons being expressed in all Shank3 isoforms. In addition, there are three alternatively spliced exons that are expressed only in tissue-specific isoforms.

The longest Shank3 isoform produces a messenger RNA (mRNA) transcript of 7,031 nucleotides, and it is expressed only in the brain and testes. mRNA is a molecule that carries genetic information from DNA to ribosomes, the cell's protein-making machinery. The Shank3 protein that is produced from the mRNA transcript is a vital component of the synapse, the junction between two neurons that allows them to communicate with each other. The protein plays a crucial role in maintaining the structure of the synapse, as well as in the regulation of the neurotransmitter signaling that takes place across the synapse.

The expression and function of the SHANK3 gene are tightly regulated by a complex series of mechanisms. One of these mechanisms is the alternative splicing of three variable exons. Alternative splicing is a process that allows different versions of a protein to be made by selecting and combining different exons. In the case of SHANK3, the selection of different exons can result in the creation of various Shank3 isoforms that have unique properties and functions.

Another mechanism that regulates SHANK3 expression is the methylation of four intragenic promoters. Methylation is a process by which a methyl group is added to the DNA molecule, which can change the way the gene is read by the cell's protein-making machinery. The methylation of intragenic promoters can affect the transcription of SHANK3, controlling the production of tissue- and time-specific isoforms of Shank3 protein.

The product of the main mRNA isoform of this gene, SH3 and multiple ankyrin repeat domains protein 3 (Shank3), is composed of 1,730 amino acids and belongs to a family of proteins that interact with receptors of the postsynaptic membrane. These multidomain proteins are important scaffolding molecules in the postsynaptic density (PSD) and function to receive and integrate synaptic signals and transduce them into postsynaptic cells. In addition to their role in the assembly of the PSD during synaptogenesis, the Shank proteins may play a role in synaptic plasticity and in the regulation of dendritic spine morphology.

Although the majority of Phelan-McDermid syndrome-associated variants are whole-gene deletions, there are a limited number of splice site, missense, nonsense, and frameshift variants that have been reported. Most individuals with SHANK3 intragenic variants are described as having autism or intellectual disability.

The genetic basis of ASD is complex, with many genes thought to be involved. One of the genes that has been linked to ASD is SHANK3, which encodes a protein that is involved in the development and function of synapses in the brain. Mutations in the SHANK3 gene have been associated with a specific type of ASD known as Phelan-McDermid syndrome (PMS).

Molecular diagnostic tests, such as Next-Generation Sequencing (NGS) and Deletion/Duplication Analysis, can be used to identify genetic variants in the SHANK3 gene that are associated with ASD. NGS allows for the simultaneous sequencing of multiple genes, providing a more comprehensive analysis of genetic variants in individuals with ASD. Deletion/Duplication Analysis is specifically designed to identify large deletions or duplications in the genetic material, which can also be associated with ASD.

The clinical utility of molecular confirmation of a clinical diagnosis is to provide a definitive diagnosis for individuals with ASD. This information can help guide decisions about treatment and management of the condition. Additionally, molecular confirmation can assist in testing at-risk relatives for specific known variants that have been identified in an affected family member.

In the case of SHANK3, molecular diagnostic tests can identify specific mutations in the gene that are associated with ASD, such as those that cause PMS. This information can be used to provide a definitive diagnosis for individuals with PMS and to guide decisions about treatment and management of the condition. Additionally, testing at-risk relatives for specific known variants can be useful in identifying individuals who may be at higher risk of developing PMS or other types of ASD.

Overall, molecular diagnostic tests such as NGS and Deletion/Duplication Analysis are important tools in the diagnosis and management of ASD and other neurodevelopmental disorders. These tests allow for the identification of specific genetic variants that are associated with these conditions, providing valuable information to patients, families, and healthcare providers.

Further research is needed to identify all the genetic factors involved and to fully understand their role in the development of autism, as well as to determine the specific environmental factors that may increase the risk for the disorder. The process of administering molecular diagnostic tests, such as Next-Generation Sequencing (NGS) and Deletion/Duplication Analysis, involves several steps.

First, a healthcare provider will typically order the test for an individual who is suspected of having a genetic condition, such as autism spectrum disorders (ASD) or a specific syndrome like Phelan-McDermid syndrome (PMS) that is associated with mutations in a specific gene, like SHANK3. The provider will collect a blood or saliva sample from the individual, which contains DNA that can be used for genetic testing.

Next, the sample is sent to a laboratory that specializes in genetic testing. At the laboratory, the DNA is extracted from the sample and purified to remove any contaminants that could interfere with the testing process.

For NGS, the purified DNA is then amplified and fragmented into small pieces. These pieces are then sequenced using a high-throughput sequencing platform. The resulting sequence data is processed using specialized software that can identify variants in the DNA sequence, such as single nucleotide variants (SNVs) or small insertions/deletions (indels), that could be associated with the condition being tested for.

For Deletion/Duplication Analysis, the purified DNA is analyzed using specialized techniques such as quantitative PCR or multiplex ligation-dependent probe amplification (MLPA). These techniques are designed to identify large deletions or duplications in the genetic material that could be associated with the condition being tested for.

In clinical settings, qPCR is widely used for the detection and quantification of infectious agents, such as bacteria and viruses, in patient samples. qPCR can be used to detect and quantify the presence of pathogenic organisms in various clinical specimens, including blood, urine, and respiratory secretions.

For example, qPCR is commonly used in the diagnosis of viral infections such as human papillomavirus (HPV), hepatitis B virus (HBV), and human immunodeficiency virus (HIV). qPCR can also be used to monitor the response to antiviral therapy and to detect drug resistance mutations.

In addition to infectious disease diagnosis, qPCR is used in cancer diagnostics to detect and quantify the presence of cancer cells or tumor markers in patient samples. qPCR can also be used to monitor the response to cancer treatment and to detect minimal residual disease (MRD), which is the presence of small amounts of cancer cells after treatment.

Multiplex Ligation-dependent Probe Amplification (MLPA) is commonly used in clinical genetics for the detection of genetic abnormalities, particularly copy number variations (CNVs). CNVs are often associated with various genetic disorders, such as autism, intellectual disability, and certain types of cancer.

In the diagnosis of genetic disorders, MLPA is used to detect the presence of CNVs in patient DNA samples. This information can be used to confirm a suspected diagnosis or to provide a diagnosis in cases where the cause of the disorder is unknown. MLPA can also be used for carrier testing and prenatal diagnosis.

In addition, MLPA can be used in cancer diagnostics to detect gene copy number changes in tumor cells. This information can be used to guide treatment decisions and to monitor the response to cancer therapy.

CNVs are structural variations in the DNA that involve the gain or loss of a specific segment of DNA. These CNVs can be caused by genetic mutations, genetic rearrangements, or chromosomal abnormalities and are often associated with various genetic disorders such as cancer, autism, and intellectual disability.

MLPA is based on the principle of hybridization and ligation of short synthetic oligonucleotide probes to specific target sequences in the DNA sample. Each probe consists of two parts, one that binds to a specific target sequence in the genome and another that can be amplified by PCR. After hybridization of the probes to the DNA sample, the probe pairs are ligated, and the ligated products are then amplified by PCR. The resulting PCR products are separated by size using capillary electrophoresis and quantified. By comparing the peak heights of the PCR products for the different probes, the copy number of the specific regions of the genome can be determined.

MLPA can analyze up to 50 different regions of the genome in a single reaction, making it a highly efficient and cost-effective method for detecting CNVs. MLPA can be used to detect CNVs in various clinical samples such as blood, saliva, and tissue samples.

MLPA has several advantages over other methods for detecting CNVs such as comparative genomic hybridization (CGH) and fluorescence in situ hybridization (FISH). MLPA is less expensive than CGH and FISH and can analyze multiple targets simultaneously. MLPA is also less labor-intensive than FISH, which requires specialized expertise and equipment.

MLPA has many applications in medical research and diagnostics. It is commonly used in clinical genetics for the detection of genetic abnormalities, particularly CNVs. MLPA can also be used in cancer diagnostics to detect gene copy number changes in tumor cells. This information can be used to guide treatment decisions and to monitor the response to cancer therapy.

Once the analysis is complete, the laboratory generates a report that summarizes the results of the testing. The report typically includes information about any variants or mutations that were identified, as well as an interpretation of the results and any recommendations for follow-up testing or medical management.

The results of these tests can be used by healthcare providers to provide a definitive diagnosis for individuals with ASD or a specific syndrome, such as PMS. This information can help guide decisions about treatment and management of the condition, as well as assist in testing at-risk relatives for specific known variants that have been identified in an affected family member.

Chromosome 22 is one of the 23 pairs of chromosomes in the human genome. It is the second smallest chromosome, with a total length of about 49 million base pairs. Chromosome 22 contains many genes that are involved in a variety of physiological processes, including those involved in development, immunity, and the regulation of gene expression.

Some of the notable genes located on chromosome 22 include SHANK3 (as previously mentioned), as well as the genes that are associated with several genetic disorders such as DiGeorge syndrome, Cat Eye syndrome, and velocardio facial syndrome.

There is also evidence that variations in certain genes on chromosome 22 may contribute to the development of psychiatric and neurodevelopmental disorders, such as schizophrenia and autism spectrum disorder.

In addition to the important genes it contains, chromosome 22 also has a substantial number of repetitive DNA sequences, including a large amount of satellite DNA, which is believed to play a role in the regulation of gene expression and the stability of the genome. Further, studies have indicated that genetic mutations associated with autism tend to cluster in certain biological pathways, such as those involved in synaptic function and communication. This provides further evidence of a genetic contribution to the disorder, as it suggests that these genetic mutations disrupt specific biological processes that are critical for normal brain development and function.

It is important to note that while the genetic component of autism is significant, environmental factors are also believed to play a role in the development of the disorder. For example, exposure to certain toxic substances during pregnancy has been linked to an increased risk for autism, and studies have also indicated that obstetrical complications, such as premature birth and low birth weight, may increase the risk for autism.

Claims about the link between ultrasound and autism have been debunked by multiple large-scale studies that have found no evidence of a causal relationship between the two. The World Health Organization, the American College of Obstetricians and Gynecologists, and the American Institute of Ultrasound in Medicine have all stated that ultrasound is safe for use during pregnancy.

Claims about a link between vaccines and autism have also been extensively studied and found to be untrue. Multiple large-scale, peer-reviewed studies have shown that vaccines do not cause autism. The Centers for Disease Control and Prevention (CDC), the World Health Organization (WHO), and the Institute of Medicine have all stated that there is no credible evidence of a causal link between vaccines and autism.

Claims about a link between 5G signals and autism are also unfounded. There is currently no evidence to suggest that 5G signals pose a risk to human health, including the development of autism. The World Health Organization and the International Commission on Non-Ionizing Radiation Protection have both stated that 5G signals are safe for human exposure.

It is important to rely on credible and evidence-based information when it comes to health and safety issues. Misinformation about the causes of autism can not only lead to unnecessary worry and fear, but it can also distract from the search for effective interventions and treatments for those with autism.

I looked up what potential medications were on the market for ASD and found this information online as I conducted a thorough investigation into the available medications on the market and obtained information from various credible sources. After reviewing the information, I personally chose not to pursue any of the options listed as they did not align with my personal beliefs and preferences. It is important to consult with a healthcare professional and make informed decisions regarding any medical treatment.

Antidepressants are commonly used to help manage depression, anxiety, and obsessive-compulsive behavior in individuals with Autism Spectrum Disorder. They work by changing the levels of certain chemicals in the brain, such as serotonin and norepinephrine, which play a role in regulating mood and behavior. However, it's important to note that the effectiveness of antidepressants can vary from person to person and side effects such as headache, nausea, and sexual dysfunction may occur.

Stimulants, such as methylphenidate (Ritalin), are sometimes used to improve focus, attention, and hyperactivity in individuals with ASD. They increase the levels of certain neurotransmitters in the brain, including dopamine and norepinephrine, which are associated with attention and motivation. The use of stimulants in individuals with ASD is still being studied and their effectiveness may vary. Common side effects include decreased appetite, trouble sleeping, and agitation.

Antipsychotics, such as risperidone (Risperdal) and aripiprazole (Abilify), are used to reduce aggressive behavior, self-injury, and irritability in some individuals with ASD. They work by blocking or reducing the effects of certain neurotransmitters in the brain, including dopamine and serotonin. Antipsychotics can have serious side effects, including weight gain, drowsiness, and increased risk of metabolic problems, and should only be used under the close supervision of a doctor.

Mood stabilizers, such as valproic acid (Depakote), are sometimes used to regulate mood swings and irritability in individuals with ASD. They work by stabilizing the levels of certain chemicals in the brain, including GABA, which is associated with regulating mood. However, mood stabilizers can have side effects, including fatigue, weight gain, and liver problems, and their effectiveness in individuals with ASD is still being studied.

It's important to keep in mind that these medications may not be effective for everyone with ASD, and the decision to use medication should be made in consultation with a doctor who specializes in treating individuals with ASD. Every individual with ASD is unique and has specific needs, and the best treatment plan will depend on the individual's symptoms and needs.

There is limited scientific evidence to support the use of CBD (cannabidiol) in treating symptoms of ASD. While some studies have shown promise in reducing anxiety, improving sleep, and reducing irritability in individuals with ASD, more research is needed to fully understand the effectiveness and safety of CBD for individuals with ASD.

It's important to note that the use of CBD is regulated differently in different countries and states, and its legal status may be unclear. In some regions, CBD products may not be approved for medical use, and their quality and composition may be unreliable.

While the limited evidence suggests that CBD may be beneficial for some individuals with ASD, it is not a substitute for comprehensive treatment and care. A comprehensive treatment plan for individuals with ASD should include a variety of evidence-based interventions, including behavioral therapy, speech and language therapy, and education and support services.

It's best to consult with a doctor who has expertise in treating individuals with ASD before considering the use of CBD. They can help determine the best treatment plan based on the individual's specific needs and medical history.

Chapter 5: Coping with ASD: Exploring Self-Medicating Strategies for Autism

If this is to be a truly scientific look into my brain function, my many knockouts and chemical drug use must be examined as well.

I have been knocked unconscious by severe blows to my head many times. There were a couple of knockouts during physical altercations, once from a pro boxer and once being hit in the back of the head with a blackjack.

There were four construction and trucking mishaps that landed me unconscious not counting the big one my TBI from the fall in 2004.

There was the time in Edmonton that I was thrown off of the football grandstand some twenty-five feet or more to the asphalt. I got up not remembering what had happened. My friend Wilf Peters witnessed the whole thing and filled me in on things later. He said that I looked up towards my aggressors and did a 'rebel yell' which was meant to mock them as I was unhurt.

I have taken LSD at dozens of times sometimes with some heavy dosages. I became unconcerned with hallucinations while under the influence of the drug for trips of several hour duration. I was taking it for a few years and then lost interest. I have picked and eaten handfuls of the tiny psychedelic psilocybin mushrooms in Vancouver and gotten high and hallucinated a few times.

Hard drugs such as heroin and cocaine held no interest for me, I am more the MMDA 'molly' speed type. I enjoyed MMDA several times but eventually lost interest.

My favorite drug is Phenmetrazine a stimulant of the central nervous system. It was previously sold under the trade name Preludin as an anorectic. Preludin has since been removed from the market. It was initially replaced by the analogue Phendimetrazine (Bontril), but this is now only rarely prescribed, due to problems with abuse. Other names that have been used for Phenmetrazine include: Defenmetrazin, Fenmetrazin, Oxazimedrine, Phenmetraline. It is by some considered to have a greater potential for addiction than the amphetamines, and has been abused in many countries, for example Sweden. When stimulant abuse first became prevalent in Sweden in the 1950s, phenmetrazine was preferred to amphetamine and methamphetamine by addicts, as it was considered the superior drug. In the autobiographical novel "*Rush*" by Kim Wozencraft, phenmetrazine is described as the most euphoric and pro-sexual of the stimulants the author used.

Unfortunately, I lost my connections for Preludin and instead have often used analogues of amyl-nitrate instead.

I concocted a memory stimulant that I used for all my university exams over many years. It involved selection of just the right ginger root at the grocery store. It had to have a head. I would buy two or three 'Head' shaped ginger roots. I used a top-of-the-line Braun juicer (I have three because of my compulsion to have spares for everything important) and would often make enough ginger juice to get me through a week or more of scheduled examinations.

With the ginger I was able to look at the blank blackboard at the front of the examination room and 'read' the answers from the professor's handwritten chalk notes. Earlier during the classes I would say to myself that I must remember what is on the board photographically and that when I took the juice later, I would re-see it during the exam. I wrote several 'A' graded exams using this technique.

I have smoked marijuana heavily since 1966. For some time in the late seventies and early eighties I smoked hashish instead of marijuana. I smoked high potency hashish heavily using several grams per day.

As I write this in 2023 cannabis has been legalized in Canada and my partner Barbara and I smoke cannabis we purchase from a legal government licenced store. We have always smoked excessively but now the pot is four or five times stronger. I prefer the sativa strains, but because she is most often the one buying, we get indica varieties in the 20% THC range.

Chapter 6: The Unique Abilities of Autistic Savants: An Insider's Perspective

Autistic savants are individuals with autism spectrum disorder (ASD) who have exceptional abilities in one or more areas, such as mathematics, music, art, or memory. These abilities, known as "islets of competence," stand in stark contrast to the individual's overall developmental or intellectual disabilities.

It is estimated that savants occur in about 10% of people with autism, and they are more commonly found in males. The exact causes of savant skills are not well understood, but research suggests that they may be related to differences in brain structure or function in individuals with autism.

I often wonder why it is that I seem to be able to learn complicated things so quickly. I think it goes far beyond having a lot of practice learning. It seems like some sort of hidden talent. For me it is the good side of ASD. I am used to having it and sometimes rely upon having the ability to learn difficult things extremely fast. I often wonder why this is possible and I enjoy taking tests, quizzes, and exams because it confirms that I must have grasped the material if I am able to score well on the tests.

I think being able to learn computer programming in my late sixties is a good example. I found it difficult conceptually at first and all of the various computer programming languages seemed very difficult to learn; but I soon caught on that it was the same thing over and over again with each new language built on precursor languages.

I also found myself to have an uncanny knack at electronic design. I have custom built many crypto-currency mining rigs using graphic cards and also purchased ASIC crypto-currency miners. Presently I am doing research loading special programs into tiny micro computers like the raspberry pi's 2040 chip and the ESP 32C2 Arduino chips that are thumbnail size. I am designing a hardware wallet for cryptographic keys.

The Canadian Security Agency (CSA) is seeking to hire individuals with mental disabilities such as Autism Spectrum Disorder (ASD), Obsessive Compulsive Disorder (OCD), Bipolar Disorder, and dyslexia. Their decision is based on the idea that individuals with these conditions may possess unique skills and abilities that could be advantageous in code breaking and encryption.

People with autism, for instance, often have exceptional attention to detail, pattern recognition skills, and the ability to focus on repetitive tasks for extended periods of time. These traits are often seen as being particularly well-suited for code breaking and encryption tasks, which require a high degree of precision and focus.

I find the fact that the CSA knows that people with ASD are good code breakers gratifying. I have been personally working on an encryption project for over a year now. The challenge is to build a small Bitcoin digital wallet that holds the owner's cryptographic keys offline. It involves secure design, avoiding outdated and compromised encryption systems like RSA and Elliptic Curves, securing chips, and networking. I find my abilities in the field somewhat surprising as I only got as far as the tenth grade in mathematics.

Similarly, individuals with OCD often have strong problem-solving skills, attention to detail, and a tendency to become deeply engrossed in repetitive tasks. These qualities can be useful in cracking complex codes and solving challenging encryption problems.

In the case of individuals with bipolar disorder, the fluctuations in their mood and energy levels can result in enhanced creativity and the ability to think outside the box, which can be beneficial in finding creative solutions to complex encryption challenges.

People with dyslexia, on the other hand, often have strong visual-spatial skills and the ability to think creatively and "outside the box". These skills can also be valuable in code breaking and encryption, as they can lead to unique approaches to solving complex problems.

It is worth noting, however, that this is not to say that individuals with these conditions are inherently better at code breaking and encryption. Rather, it is the unique skills and abilities that some individuals with these conditions possess that make them an asset to the CSA in these areas.

It is also important to emphasize that the CSA is committed to promoting diversity and inclusion, and that the agency recognizes the unique skills and abilities that individuals with disabilities can bring to the workplace. By seeking to hire more individuals with disabilities, the CSA aims to create a more inclusive and diverse work environment, where individuals of all abilities can thrive and contribute to the agency's success.

People with ASD have certain cognitive abilities and traits that can make them well-suited to advanced computer programming and coding. Their attention to detail is a crucial skill in computer programming, where even small errors can cause significant problems. Their strong pattern recognition skills and ability to focus for long periods of time also make them well-suited for coding, where a high level of focus and pattern recognition are important.

Additionally, people with ASD often think in a systematic, organized manner, which can help them understand complex programming concepts and algorithms. Some individuals with autism also have strong visual-spatial skills, which can be an asset in computer programming where visualizing code and abstract concepts is important.

Furthermore, people with ASD often prefer routine and predictability, which makes coding an ideal choice as it involves following a set of rules and structures. These abilities and traits, when combined with proper support and resources, can make individuals with autism excel in computer programming and coding.

Famous individuals who have been diagnosed with, or have self-reported having, ASD include Elon Musk, CEO of Tesla, SpaceX, Neuralink, and The Boring Company. Temple Grandin is another famous individual with autism, she is an animal scientist and author known for her work in improving the welfare of livestock. Satoshi Tajiri, the creator of the Pokémon franchise, is also believed to be on the autism spectrum.

In the entertainment industry, Dan Aykroyd, an actor and comedian best known for his role in the Ghostbusters franchise, and Tim Burton, a film director and producer known for his visually stunning and quirky films such as Edward Scissorhands and Alice in Wonderland, are also believed to be on the autism spectrum. Darrell Hammond, a comedian and impressionist best known for his long-standing role on Saturday Night Live, is another individual who is known to have autism.

Susan Boyle, the singer who rose to international fame after appearing on Britain's Got Talent, and Michael Fitzgerald, a clinical professor of child and adolescent psychiatry at Trinity College Dublin, are believed to have autism. Finally, Andy Warhol, the artist considered one of the most important figures in the pop art movement, is another well-known individual who is believed to have had autism.

It's important to note that not all of these individuals have been diagnosed with autism by a medical professional, and that self-reported diagnoses should be viewed with caution. However, these individuals have spoken publicly about their experiences with autism or have been identified by others as having traits commonly associated with the condition.

It is difficult to definitively diagnose historical figures with ASD as the condition was only first described in the 1940s and diagnostic criteria have changed over time. However, some people believe that some historical figures may have had traits associated with autism.

Albert Einstein, the physicist known for his theories of special and general relativity, is often considered as a possible individual with autism. Einstein was known for his intense focus and attention to detail, as well as his difficulty with social interactions. Albert Einstein: known for his exceptional intelligence and contribution to science, but he struggled with communication.

Isaac Newton, the mathematician and physicist known for his work on the laws of motion and universal gravitation, is also often considered as a possible individual with autism. Newton was known for his intense focus and solitary lifestyle, as well as his difficulty with people. He was considered as one of the greatest scientists of all time but was known for his introverted personality and poor social skills.

Nikola Tesla, despite his numerous contributions to science and technology was known for his difficulty in forming close relationships and socializing. Tesla's erratic behaviour is indicative of a person with ASD.

Wolfgang Amadeus Mozart, the composer and musician known for his prolific output of classical music, is another individual who is believed to have had autism. He was known for his introverted personality and difficulty in socializing with others.

Hans Christian Andersen, the Danish author best known for his fairy tales, is also believed to have had autism. Andersen was known for his imaginative and vivid storytelling and his reclusive personality and difficulty in forming close relationships with others.

It is important to note that these individuals have not been diagnosed with autism by a medical professional and that their diagnosis is based on anecdotal accounts and observations of their behavior and traits. However, these individuals have been identified by some as having traits commonly associated with autism.

There are several well-known business leaders who have publicly disclosed having ASD , including:

1. Bill Gates, co-founder of Microsoft
2. Larry Ellison, co-founder of Oracle Corporation
3. Mark Zuckerberg, co-founder of Facebook
4. Satoshi Tajiri, creator of Pokémon
5. Elon Musk

Paranoia is not a defining characteristic of ASD. While some individuals with ASD may experience paranoia, it is not a symptom commonly associated with the condition. Each person with ASD is unique and may experience a range of symptoms and behaviors. It is important to understand that paranoia is not a symptom that is specific to individuals with ASD and can occur in people with or without the condition.

Chapter 7: Accessing Support: Navigating Insurance Coverage for ASD Treatment

Insurance coverage for the treatment of ASD varies depending on the type of insurance and the country or state in which the individual resides. In many countries, including the United States, insurance companies are required by law to provide coverage for the diagnosis and treatment of certain medical conditions, including autism.

In the United States, under the Affordable Care Act (ACA), private insurance plans and Medicaid are required to provide coverage for the diagnosis and treatment of autism, including behavioral therapy, speech and language therapy, and medication management. However, the specifics of coverage, such as the extent of coverage and the types of services covered, can vary depending on the insurance plan.

In Canada, under the Canada Health Act, all Canadian citizens and permanent residents have access to medically necessary hospital and physician services, which includes coverage for the diagnosis and treatment of autism.

In 2004 I took a fall at work and hit my head. As described in greater detail in a chapter later in this book I was on compensation for nearly two and a half years related to my TBI and was fully covered first by the Manitoba Workman's Compensation Board and then by wage loss coverage from Standard Life.

In other countries, such as the United Kingdom, autism is considered a disability, and individuals with autism are eligible for support and services through the National Health Service (NHS).

It's best to check with the specific insurance provider to determine the coverage for ASD, as well as to understand any limitations and exclusions that may apply. A doctor or a specialist in the treatment of autism can also provide guidance on insurance options and coverage.

There is limited evidence to suggest that individuals with ASD are at a higher risk of criminal incarceration. However, it is important to note that the relationship between autism and criminal behavior is complex and influenced by many factors, including co-occurring mental health conditions, access to appropriate education and support services, and social and economic factors.

Studies have shown that individuals with autism may be more likely to engage in behaviors that can lead to criminal justice involvement, such as wandering from safe environments, impulsivity, and difficulty with communication and social interaction. However, these behaviors are often a result of the challenges faced by individuals with autism and are not necessarily indicative of criminal intent.

There is a lack of comprehensive data on the prevalence of criminal justice involvement among individuals with autism, but some estimates suggest that the rate of incarceration among individuals with autism may be higher than the general population.

To reduce the risk of criminal justice involvement for individuals with autism, it is important to provide access to appropriate education and support services, such as behavioral therapy, speech and language therapy, and educational and vocational programs. This can help individuals with autism develop the skills and supports needed to successfully navigate their communities and reduce the risk of criminal justice involvement.

It is also important to provide law enforcement and criminal justice professionals with education and training on the unique needs and challenges faced by individuals with autism. This can help ensure that individuals with autism are treated with respect and dignity, and that their rights are protected, regardless of whether they encounter the criminal justice system.

Chapter 8: ASD and the World of Music, Video Games, and Sports: Finding a Place to Thrive

Individuals with ASD can play video games. In fact, many individuals with autism enjoy playing video games and find them to be a fun and engaging form of entertainment.

Video games can also provide therapeutic benefits for individuals with autism. For example, some video games can help improve social skills, communication skills, and problem-solving skills. Video games can also provide an opportunity for individuals with autism to practice coping strategies, such as managing emotions and handling stressful situations.

However, it's important to note that not all video games are appropriate for individuals with autism. Some video games may contain violent or mature content that is not suitable for individuals with autism. It's also important to be mindful of the amount of time spent playing video games, as excessive gaming can lead to social isolation.

Individuals with ASD can have varied interests and preferences, including music. Some individuals with autism enjoy listening to music and may have a particular interest in a specific genre or type of music.

Music can also have therapeutic benefits for individuals with autism. For example, music can help improve communication skills, social skills, and emotional regulation. Music therapy is a form of therapy that uses music to address physical, emotional, cognitive, and social needs of individuals with autism.

However, not all individuals with autism have an interest in music, and some may even have an aversion to certain types of music. It's important to be mindful of the individual's preferences and to respect their decisions about what they do and do not enjoy.

Individuals with ASD can have varied interests and preferences, including sports. Some individuals with autism enjoy watching sports and may have a particular interest in a specific sport or team. Watching sports can provide an opportunity for individuals with autism to develop social skills, such as communicating with others about sports and engaging in friendly competition. It can also provide a form of entertainment and a way to relieve stress.

However, not all individuals with autism have an interest in sports, and some may even have an aversion to certain types of sports or physical activities. It's important to be mindful of the individual's preferences and to respect their decisions about what they do and do not enjoy.

Individuals with ASD can have strong connections with animals, particularly cats. It is not uncommon for individuals with autism to have a fondness for animals, including cats, and to form strong bonds with them.

There are several reasons why individuals with autism may have a special connection with cats. Firstly, cats can provide comfort and emotional support, which can be particularly important for individuals with autism who may struggle with social interactions and emotional regulation. Cats are also generally low-maintenance and can be independent, which can be appealing to individuals with autism who may prefer solitary activities.

Additionally, cats can provide a calming and soothing presence, which can help reduce anxiety and stress levels for individuals with autism. The repetitive and predictable behavior of cats can also be comforting for individuals with autism, who may struggle with processing sensory information and experiencing sensory overload.

However, it's important to note that not all individuals with autism have an interest in animals, including cats. Some individuals with autism may have an aversion to animals or may not be comfortable around them. It's important to respect the individual's preferences and to be mindful of their comfort level with animals.

ASD affects individuals of all races, ethnicities, and socioeconomic backgrounds, and both males and females.

Studies have shown that the incidence of autism is consistent across races and ethnicities, with the prevalence of autism being higher in white and non-Hispanic populations. However, cultural attitudes towards autism, access to healthcare, and misdiagnosis or underdiagnosis of autism can impact the identification and diagnosis of autism in different racial and ethnic groups.

In terms of sex, autism is four to five times more likely to be diagnosed in males than females, with a male to female ratio of 4:1. This disparity is thought to be due to a combination of biological, diagnostic, and cultural factors, including differences in the presentation of autism symptoms in males and females, and gender biases in the diagnostic process.

Research into the causes and risk factors for autism is ongoing, and it is important to note that no one factor can predict the likelihood of developing autism. It is a complex disorder with multiple causes, including genetic and environmental factors.

It's important to raise awareness about autism and to promote early identification and treatment, regardless of race, ethnicity, or sex, to ensure that individuals with autism receive the support and resources they need to lead fulfilling lives.

Chapter 9: Finding Help: Organizations and Resources for Individuals with ASD

ASD is a complex disorder that affects individuals of all ages, and support from organizations and communities can play a vital role in helping individuals with autism and their families. There are many national autism support groups that offer a variety of resources and services, including information and advocacy, support groups, educational programs, and a platform for individuals with autism and their families to connect with others and share their experiences.

Here are some of the national autism support groups:

1. Autism Speaks: This organization is dedicated to promoting solutions across the spectrum and throughout the life span for individuals with autism and their families. They offer a range of resources, including information and advocacy, support services, and research.

2. The Autism Society of America: This organization is dedicated to improving the lives of all affected by autism by increasing public awareness, advocacy, and providing resources and services to individuals with autism and their families.

3. The Autistic Self Advocacy Network (ASAN): This organization is run by and for Autistic individuals and provides support, resources, and advocacy for the Autistic community.

4. National Autistic Association (NAA): This organization is dedicated to supporting families affected by autism, providing information and resources, and advocating for the needs of individuals with autism and their families.

5. Association for Science in Autism Treatment (ASAT): This organization is dedicated to promoting evidence-based treatment for individuals with autism and providing accurate information about autism to families and professionals.

6. The Arc: This organization is dedicated to promoting and protecting the human rights of people with intellectual and developmental disabilities, including autism.

7. Talk About Curing Autism (TACA): This organization provides support and information to families affected by autism, including support groups, educational programs, and a resource center.

8. Generation Rescue: This organization provides hope, help, and healing to families affected by autism through research, education, and support.

9. National Council on Severe Autism: This organization provides support and resources to families of individuals with severe autism, including information on treatment and support services.

10. Autism Science Foundation (ASF): This organization is dedicated to supporting and promoting autism research by providing funding and other resources to scientists and organizations working in the field of autism.

Each of these organizations offers a unique set of resources and services, and it's important to research and evaluate the specific goals and services offered by each organization to determine which one best meets your needs and interests. Consulting with a doctor or a specialist in the treatment of autism can also be helpful in determining which resources and support groups may be most beneficial for you.

Here are some Autism Spectrum Disorder (ASD) support groups in Canada:

1. Autism Canada: This organization provides information, support, and advocacy for individuals with autism and their families.
2. The Canadian Autism Spectrum Disorders Alliance (CASDA): This organization is dedicated to improving the lives of individuals with autism by promoting awareness, advocacy, and providing support and resources to families.
3. The Autistic Community in Ontario (ACO): This organization provides support, resources, and advocacy for Autistic individuals and their families in Ontario.
4. The Saskatchewan Asperger's Disorder Association (SADA): This organization provides support and resources for individuals with Asperger's syndrome and their families in Saskatchewan.
5. The British Columbia Autism Association (BCAA): This organization provides support, resources,

and advocacy for individuals with autism and their families in British Columbia.

6. Quebec Autism Foundation: This organization provides support and resources for individuals with autism and their families in Quebec.

7. Autism Support Network: This organization provides support, resources, and advocacy for individuals with autism and their families across Canada.

8. The Autism Network for Dietary Intervention (ANDI): This organization provides support and resources for families of individuals with autism who are following a gluten-free, casein-free (GFCF) diet.

9. Talk About Curing Autism (TACA) Canada: This organization provides support, resources, and advocacy for families affected by autism in Canada.

10. Autism Ontario: This organization provides support, resources, and advocacy for individuals with autism and their families in Ontario.

Personally, I have always felt that the best advice online is the 'Autism from the Inside' YouTube channel with Paul Micallef and all the help that he offers subscribers.

Paul has lived the life of an aspie and is willing to share his experiences and he offers some solutions and better ways to view the world for anyone with ASD.

Chapter 10: My Journey to Diagnosis: Personal Reflections on Clinical Examinations for ASD

-

- Actual report 1994

Summary and Recommendations.

Jeremiah Coffey is a 45-year-old man seen for neuropsychological assessment to determine whether he shows a pattern of cognitive strengths and deficits which would be consistent with a learning disability. Assessment of Mr. Coffey's general cognitive ability indicates a significant split between his verbal skills, which lie in the <u>superior</u> range, and his nonverbal skills, which lie in the <u>average</u> range. In keeping with this observed split, specific tests for verbal fluency and naming were in the high to superior ranges. Given those skills, it is also not surprising that Mr. Coffey's academic performance was found to be beyond grade 12 levels for all areas but arithmetic. Where grade-equivalent scores fell at the beginning of grade 11. Mr. Coffey is tended to perform in the average range on specific tests of visual- perceptual, visio-spatial, constructive and motor skills, which is consistent with his average performance on the nonverbal component of the general test of cognitive ability. Performance on tests of attention were variable, but also tended to fall in the average range. Memory for nonverbal materials fell in the average to superior ranges and memory. Related verbal material was average. The only significant impairments noted during the testing were in new learning of lists of verbal material and in one test of a motor skill.

Mr. Coffey is evidencing a significant split in his verbal and nonverbal skills. Likely this relatively poorer ability to carry out tasks requiring spatial planning and execution is what he is seeing when he experiences himself as less able to coordinate his movements and plan physical things. With the exception of results on one motor task for one hand Mr. Coffey's skills in these areas, however, are roughly in the average range. As such, these results while suggesting a relative deficit in nonverbal skills compared with the very strong verbal skills would not explain his difficulties in elementary school and high school.

It should be also noted that Mr. Coffey's strongest scores are in tests which are heavily reliant on overlearned material. (vocabulary, general knowledge, etc,). Quite likely these results are a product of Mr. Coffey's exceptional efforts to learn, and his recognition of his relatively greater strengths in verbal reasoning. He indicated in our interview with him that he has been reading upwards of six hours a day for years and he spends an inordinate amount of time mastering difficult written material because he feels this is where he can excel.

Difficulties with new learning evidenced in the present testing are quite germane to Mr. Coffey's struggles with his education and possibly his efforts to enter law school. Results of testing show a large gap between Mr. Coffey's store of overlearned words and facts, and his ability to learn novel material, especially if it's presented free of context. Even within the context of a meaningful paragraph Mr. Coffey's ability to memorize material is only average. Quite likely what is happening is that Mr. Coffey has above average skills in verbal reasoning, is able to store verbal information and retrieve it from memory given enough time and effort. And he has exceptionally good learning strategies but essentially, he has a poor memory. His superior scores and verbally loaded tests are thus the product of his incredible efforts to learn and his ability to work with verbal motor material. His ability to work with verbal material once it is memorized. In a similar vein as early childhood, difficulties can be understood as his struggle to learn with impaired memory at a time due to his developing compensatory skills. Essentially, he has a poor memory.

The pattern of results observed during the present testing are consistent with the memory defect and significantly poorer spatial than verbal ability. Usually, the diagnosis of learning disability is made on the basis of significant differences in performance on tests of academic ability. Clearly Mr. Coffey is not showing differential responses on such tests. However, in Mr. Coffey's case, his efforts at compensating for his poor memory have elevated his basic knowledge to the point that tests tapping over learned material are unlikely to note any differential effects. Further, Mr. Coffey's difficulties do not lie in the areas of learning usually considered to be where making a diagnosis of learning disabilities such as reading, writing and arithmetic, although his memory problems have. Likely the difficulties in these areas in the past a memory difficult to the kind of observed during testing. However, as likely had profound impact on Mr. Coffey's potential to learn from his this perspective, it is our considered opinion that Mr. Coffey has learning problems. If not a learning disability, though of unclear etiology, given his long standing and early academic difficulties, his difficulties are most likely developmental in nature.

Given Mr. Coffey strong cognitive report performance, there is no need for him to undergo repeat neuro psychological assessment in the future, however, we would please to be Mr. Coffey again if clinically indicated. Thank you for this referral if there are any questions regarding this success, but please do not. Hesitate to contact Dr. Mirna Vrbancic Ph.D. Registered Psychologist Supervisor at the Department of Clinical Health Psychology. Royal University Hospital Saskatoon, Saskatchewan

---

*actual report 2004

Dear Dr. Hobbs,

Thank you for referring this 55-year-old righthanded man who presents with a concussion.

Mr. Coffey describes working inside his semi truck May 30th. And the next thing he realized was lying on the ground beside it with an occipital scalp contusion and laceration. He does not recollect how he fell but surmises that he had left the door ajar and upon attempting to support himself on the door, he fell out and hit his head. He felt his jaw displaced, and upon manipulating it, he says the pain made him blackout once more. He was unable to get up for some time, although eventually he got up on his own and walked to the office.

Since then, he has had difficulty concentrating, headache, dizziness/ imbalance, all recently significantly improved. He denies any past history of seizures or blackouts otherwise.

His examination and investigations in the emergency department were otherwise normal or negative. Overall, he feels fairly well, and denies any underlying or background cognitive difficulties or behavioral problems. No collateral history was available. He does say that he naps more frequently, attributing this to his lifestyle. He describes chronic mild apraxia [1] (dyslexia, according to him). He denies any taste or smell changes [2], nor any other focal [3] or neurological problems.

Medical history. Relatively healthy. Weight gain over the past year. Non-smoker. No alcohol or drugs.

Medications. Ginkgo biloba. Melatonin. Green tea extract. Various other supplementals, vitamins, minerals.

Family history. Not well known. Unremarkable.

Examination. Alert. Oriented. No distress. Flatter effect. [4] somewhat vague historian with occasional tangential thinking. Dressed in summer shirt with cartoon action figure, bold jewelry. Speech and language otherwise intact. Mild to moderate praxis difficulty. (Luria test) Word lists starting with letter F reasonable. animal lists excellent. Digit span [5] excellent. Registration good [6], recall 1/3 with cueing. improved to 3/3 on 2nd questioning. Clock drawing almost 4/4. (Incorrect arm lengths, corrected when pointed out.) initial difficulty with diagram copying. Pupils equal and reactive and visual fields full. Funduscopy [7] unremarkable. Olfactory sense was not objectively normal. No cranial nerve abnormalities were otherwise identified. There was no arm drift, and his tone, strength, and coordination in his upper and lower extremities was normal. His reflexes were grade two to two plus upper extremities, grade two plus to three lower [8], with downgoing planters bilaterally. [9] He had subtle. palmomental and glabellar tap reflexes [10] and relatively easy to elicit snout reflex. [11] Romberg sign [12] was not present and his gait, stance including heel, toe, tandem walking was normal. No postural instability was identified.

Impression. Regarding the episode itself. It is impossible to determine. The actual etiology. Although cardiac and primary neurologic problems need to be excluded. I'm ordering an MRI. And an EEG Certainly the symptoms. Which now have improved. Are consistent with post concussive syndrome. However, I am unclear regarding. Some possible underlying cognitive compromise. Possibly frontal, temporal $_{13}$. I'll interview his wife at the next visit. In the meantime, I have advised him to refrain from driving. Thank you again for the referral and please contact me with any further questions.

Stefan Pacin , MD, FRCPC neurology. 07/15/2004

*Actual report   2004

Dear doctor Hobbs.

I saw Mr. Coffey again today September 27th, 2004, accompanied by his wife. Again, he comes across as somewhat tangential [14], And he continues to describe concentration difficulties and apraxia (Although. Last time he said that the concussive symptoms had markedly improved.) His wife also gives the example suggesting he has declining executive dysfunction as well as apraxia. There was no concrete description of personality changes although they both describe his symptom onset after his fall. The MRI does not demonstrate any shear injury, although it does show generalized atrophy.

Mr. Coffey may well have a neurodegenerative process frontal, temporal or Alzheimer's. Which he has been successfully compensating for some time. Their recent head injury. May have brought out his symptoms more (partial decompensation) Although he has improved. The etiology of his blackout is still uncertain. And I'm ordering a repeat EEG sleep deprived [15]. I have also ordered some blood work to help exclude secondary causes of cognitive dysfunction. Nuro, psychological evaluation. And I will see him again after his, EEG.

Stefan Pacin M.D. FRCPC Neurology

Explanation of some of the terms used by Dr. Pacin and my comment.

1. A praxis difficulty, also known as apraxia, can be diagnosed through various tests, including the Luria test. The Luria test is a neuropsychological assessment used to evaluate a person's ability to plan and execute complex motor movements. It involves asking the individual to perform various tasks, such as imitating gestures or actions, constructing objects with building blocks, or using tools.

In the context of autism, a diagnosis of praxis difficulty by a neurologist may indicate the presence of autism spectrum disorder. Research has shown that some individuals with autism experience difficulties with motor planning and coordination, which can manifest as apraxia. However, it is important to note that not all individuals with autism will have praxis difficulties, and not all individuals with praxis difficulties will have autism.

Apraxia is a motor disorder characterized by difficulty planning and executing voluntary movements, even though the individual has the physical ability to do so. It can be classified into different types, depending on the specific movements affected and the underlying cause of the disorder.

Some examples of apraxia include:

- Ideomotor apraxia: difficulty performing gestures or movements in response to verbal commands, such as waving goodbye or making a fist.
- Ideational apraxia: difficulty planning and coordinating movements necessary to complete a task, such as buttoning a shirt or using utensils.
- Limb-kinetic apraxia: difficulty with fine motor movements, such as writing or tying shoelaces.

In the context of autism, apraxia may be indicative of the condition in some individuals, as some research has shown that individuals with autism experience difficulties with motor planning and coordination.

A diagnosis of apraxia is typically made by a neurologist, who will perform a series of tests to assess the individual's ability to plan and execute movements. These tests may include the Luria test, which involves asking the individual to perform specific tasks, such as imitating gestures or using tools. The neurologist may also assess the individual's muscle strength, coordination, and reflexes to rule out other potential causes of motor difficulties.

---

2. Dr. Pacin asked me to sniff an unknown substance in a small tin. I could not smell anything. He said it was coffee and everyone should know the smell of coffee. I pointed out to him that he was using very stale old dry coffee grounds for the test which had

lost its characteristic "wake up and smell the coffee" aroma. He agreed to another test. He rattled something in another small tin. He asked me to sniff and removed it from under my nose. He asked me what it was, and I said Chiclets' gum. He laughed. Its cloves. Everyone knows cloves. I said what are cloves. I have no idea what cloves are or how they smell.

---

3. In addition to apraxia, individuals with autism may also experience other focal or neurological problems. Seizures are common among individuals with autism, with approximately one-third of individuals with autism also having epilepsy. Sensory Processing Disorders are also common, where individuals may experience sensory sensitivities or difficulties processing sensory information such as sounds, smells, or touch.

Movement Disorders may also be present in individuals with autism, such as clumsiness, tremors, or tics. Attention Deficit Hyperactivity Disorder (ADHD) is also commonly co-occurring with autism, where individuals may experience inattention, impulsiveness, and hyperactivity. Executive Functioning Difficulties, such as difficulties with planning, prioritizing, and carrying out tasks, may also be present in individuals with autism.

---

4. Flat affect refers to a lack of emotional expressiveness or limited emotional range. In other words, individuals with flat affect may not display typical emotional responses such as facial expressions, tone of voice, or body language, which are important for conveying emotions and building social connections. This trait is commonly associated with individuals with Autism Spectrum Disorder (ASD). People with ASD may struggle with understanding and expressing emotions, which can lead to a flat affect. However, it is important to note that flat affect is not present in all individuals with ASD, and some individuals may show a full range of emotions. Overall, flat affect can impact social interactions and communication for individuals with ASD, but with support and treatment, they can improve their emotional expressiveness and build stronger social connections.

---

5. The Digit Span test is a commonly used neuropsychological test that assesses an individual's short-term memory and attention span. It is often used as part of a larger battery of tests to diagnose various neurological or psychological conditions, including autism, ADHD, and dementia.

In the Digit Span test, the individual is asked to listen to a series of numbers (usually ranging from 2 to 9) and then repeat them back in the same order. The number of digits the individual can correctly recall is recorded, and the test is typically repeated with increasing numbers of digits to assess the individual's ability to hold and process information in their short-term memory. The results of the Digit Span test can provide important information about an individual's cognitive abilities, including their attention span, working memory, and ability to process and recall information. It can also help identify specific difficulties or strengths in these areas, which can be useful in making a diagnosis and developing an appropriate treatment plan.

---

6. Registration in a neurological evaluation refers to the process of recording information or stimuli into an individual's memory. It is an important component of many neuropsychological tests, as it measures an individual's ability to process, store, and recall information.

During a registration task, the individual is presented with a series of stimuli, such as words, letters, numbers, or images. The individual is then asked to recall as many of the stimuli as they can, either immediately after presentation or after a delay. The number of stimuli that the individual can correctly recall is recorded and used as an indicator of their memory function.

Registration is often used in combination with other neuropsychological tests to assess an individual's memory and attention abilities, as well as to identify specific difficulties or strengths in these areas. For example, an individual with a deficit in registration may have trouble retaining information, even if they can comprehend and process it correctly.

---

7. Funduscopy is an examination of the interior surface of the eye, including the retina, blood vessels, and optic disk. It is typically performed using an ophthalmoscope, which is a handheld device that shines a light into the eye to allow the examiner to see the interior structures of the eye.

Funduscopy is an important diagnostic tool in ophthalmology and neurology, as it can reveal information about the health of the eye and the health of the central nervous system. For example, funduscopy can reveal changes in the blood vessels, optic disk, or retina that may indicate conditions such as glaucoma, diabetic retinopathy, or a stroke.

It is important to note that funduscopy is a non-invasive examination and typically causes no discomfort or pain. However, in some cases, anesthetic drops may be used to dilate the pupil for a more thorough examination.

8. The evaluation of the individual's reflexes involved testing the knee-jerk reflex, which is a measure of the body's automatic response to a sudden stimulus. The reflex is graded on a scale of 0 to 4, with 4 being the strongest reflex and 0 being no reflex present.

In this case, the results of the reflex evaluation indicated that the individual's reflexes in their upper extremities were rated as a grade 2 to 2 plus, which means that their reflexes were slightly above average. In their lower extremities, their reflexes were rated as a grade 2 plus to 3, which indicates that their reflexes were average to slightly above average.

A grade 2 reflex is characterized by a moderate, brisk response. This means that when the knee-jerk reflex is tested, the individual's leg will kick out in a noticeable and fairly strong manner.

A grade 3 reflex is considered to be strong and overactive. When tested, the individual's leg will kick out very quickly and strongly.

A grade 2 plus reflex is between a grade 2 and a grade 3, meaning that the reflex is above average but not quite as strong as a grade 3 reflex. I find the results puzzling because I thought that being fast at most things would give me faster than normal reflexes.

---

9. The results also indicated that the individual had downgoing plantar reflexes bilaterally, meaning that the individual's toes curl downward when the bottom of their foot is stimulated. During the test, the healthcare provider stimulates the sole of the foot by gently stroking it from the heel to the toes. In a normal response, the toes curl downward (flexion) in response to the stimulus. This is known as a negative or normal response. However, in certain neurological conditions or brain damage, an abnormal response known as a positive Babinski sign may occur.

A positive Babinski sign is characterized by the extension (upward movement) of the big toe and sometimes the spreading of the other toes. This abnormal response suggests dysfunction or damage to the corticospinal tract, particularly the upper motor neurons originating from the brain.

Brain damage can occur due to various factors, such as traumatic brain injury, stroke, tumors, or infections. When these conditions affect the corticospinal tract, the Plan Tar Reflex can provide valuable information about potential damage or dysfunction.

---

10. Palmomental and glabellar tap reflexes are tests used in a neurological examination to assess the function of the central nervous system. The palmomental reflex is tested by tapping the thenar eminence of the hand while the individual is asked to keep their eyes closed. The thenar muscles are three short muscles located at the base of the thumb. The muscle bellies produce a bulge, known as the thenar eminence. They are responsible for the fine movements of the thumb.

The glabellar tap reflex is tested by gently tapping the patient's forehead between the eyebrows with a reflex hammer. The resulting muscle responses and reflexes can provide information about the state of the central nervous system and can help in diagnosing conditions such as brain injuries, neurodegenerative diseases, and other neurological disorders.

---

11. The Snout test is a simple but useful tool in the neurological examination. It is performed by asking the patient to perform specific facial movements that assess the function of the facial nerve, also known as the seventh cranial nerve. The facial nerve is responsible for controlling the muscles of facial expression, and damage to this nerve can result in weakness or paralysis of these muscles, leading to changes in facial appearance and difficulty with certain facial movements.

During the Snout test, the patient is asked to wrinkle their forehead, close their eyes tightly, and puff out their cheeks. The clinician assesses the strength and symmetry of these movements, as well as any drooping or asymmetry of the mouth or eye. These movements allow for assessment of the upper and lower divisions of the facial nerve, which control different groups of muscles.

Abnormalities in the Snout test can indicate various neurological conditions, such as a Bell's palsy, a facial nerve injury from head trauma, or a brainstem lesion. It can also provide information about the location and extent of the nerve damage, which can be useful in developing a treatment plan.

---

12. The Romberg sign is a clinical test used to assess a person's ability to maintain balance and stability. It is used to evaluate the function of the sensory systems, particularly the proprioception system, which is responsible for providing information about the body's position in space.

The test is performed by asking the person to stand with their feet together and arms at their sides, with their eyes open. They are then asked to close their eyes and maintain their balance. If the person sways or falls, it is considered a positive Romberg sign, which indicates a problem with the sensory system.

A positive Romberg sign can indicate a variety of conditions, including peripheral neuropathy, which is a type of nerve damage that affects the peripheral nervous system. It can also be a sign of conditions such as spinal cord injury, multiple sclerosis, or vestibular disorders, which affect the inner ear and balance.

---

13. The frontal and temporal lobes are two of the four main lobes of the brain and play a crucial role in cognitive function. They are responsible for a variety of functions such as decision making, problem solving, planning, controlling movement, processing auditory information, language, and memory.

Damage to the frontal and temporal lobes can result in a range of neurological conditions and symptoms, such as executive dysfunction, language problems, memory impairment, hearing loss, and more. For example, frontal lobe damage can result in executive dysfunction syndrome, which is characterized by problems with decision making, planning, and problem solving. Temporal lobe damage can result in conditions such as aphasia, which is a language disorder, or amnesia, which is a memory impairment.

According to studies, approximately 50% of all traumatic brain injuries (TBIs) result in damage to the frontal and temporal lobes. In the United States, TBI is a leading cause of death and disability, and it is estimated that 2.5 million people sustain a TBI each year. In addition, conditions such as stroke, dementia, and neurodegenerative disorders can also result in damage to the frontal and temporal lobes.

---

14. Tangential thinking refers to the tendency to move away from the main topic of conversation or thought to another unrelated topic. This type of behavior is common in individuals with ASD and is often referred to as "tangentiality." People with ASD may have difficulty staying on topic and following a linear train of thought, leading them to jump from one idea to another without clear connections between them. This can make communication and social interactions challenging, but with support and understanding, individuals with ASD can learn to better control and manage their tangential thinking.

---

15. An EEG (electroencephalogram) is a test that measures the electrical activity of the brain. A regular EEG is typically performed when the person is awake and alert, whereas a sleep-deprived EEG is performed after the person has been kept awake for an extended period of time, usually overnight.

The main difference between the two is the level of brain activity. During a regular EEG, the brain is typically more active, producing a higher frequency of electrical signals. In contrast, during a sleep-deprived EEG, the brain is less active, producing a lower frequency of electrical signals.

Sleep deprivation can impact brain activity and highlight certain neurological conditions, such as epilepsy, that may not be as evident during a regular EEG. Additionally, the results of a sleep-deprived EEG can provide valuable information about sleep patterns and help diagnose sleep disorders.

Glucose, a simple sugar, is the primary energy source for all cells in the body. The brain, being rich in neurons, is the most metabolically demanding organ, consuming about half of the glucose energy in the body. Brain functions, including memory, learning, and thinking, are closely linked to glucose levels and the brain's efficient use of this fuel source. A lack of glucose in the brain can disrupt the production of neurotransmitters, leading to a breakdown in communication between neurons. Hypoglycemia, a common complication of diabetes resulting from low blood glucose levels, can deprive the brain of energy, leading to poor cognitive function and attention.

Dr. Vera Novak, an associate professor of medicine at Beth Israel Deaconess Medical Center, emphasizes the brain's dependence on glucose as its primary energy source, as it cannot function without it. However, excessive glucose consumption can be detrimental to brain health. Animal studies have linked fructose consumption to cellular aging and excessive glucose intake to memory and cognitive deficiencies. Brain positron emission tomography (PET) is a diagnostic imaging technique that allows medical professionals to visualize and measure the metabolic activity of the brain. The test involves the injection of a small amount of a radioactive substance, known as a tracer, into the patient's bloodstream. The tracer is then transported by the blood to the brain, where it accumulates in areas of high metabolic activity.

Glucose, a simple sugar, is one of the most commonly used tracers in brain PET imaging. When glucose is absorbed by the brain cells, it undergoes a series of metabolic processes that produce energy to fuel the brain's functions. In PET imaging, a radioactive isotope of glucose, known as fluorodeoxyglucose (FDG), is used as a tracer. Once injected into the bloodstream, FDG is transported to the brain and accumulates in areas of high glucose metabolism. The tracer emits small amounts of radiation that can be detected by a PET scanner, producing images that reflect the brain's metabolic activity.

Brain PET scans are valuable tools for diagnosing and monitoring a range of neurological conditions, including Alzheimer's disease, Parkinson's disease, epilepsy, and brain tumors. The test provides detailed information about the metabolic activity of different regions of the brain, allowing doctors to detect changes in brain function and identify areas of abnormal activity or damage.

The test accurately details the size, shape, and see in real-time the functioning of the brain. Unlike other scans, a brain PET scan allows doctors a view of not only the structure of the brain, but how it's functioning as well.
Positron emission tomography (PET) scans are a valuable diagnostic tool that utilizes biochemical processes to study bodily functions. One of the significant advantages of PET scans is their ability to detect diseases before the symptoms and signs appear, making them more effective compared to other imaging tests.

Moreover, PET imaging can be used as an alternative to biopsy and other exploratory surgeries to determine how far a disease has spread since it studies metabolic functions of a patient. PET scans can differentiate between non-cancerous and cancerous tumors, making them the most precise medical tools to help minimize the number of unnecessary surgeries due to wrong staging data and diagnosis.

PET scans are also useful for diagnosing early stages of certain neurological illnesses, such as Alzheimer's disease, epilepsy, and other mental illnesses. Another benefit of PET scans is that they are the best options for people who are afraid of getting infections from medical procedures.

Compared to other forms of CT scans, PET scans are safer since the radiation dosage one is exposed to is relatively low. In summary, PET scans offer a range of benefits, including their precision in diagnosing diseases, safety, and ability to detect diseases before symptoms appear.

Chapter 11: Understanding Psychological Testing: A Guide to Different Types of Assessments

The Law School Admission Test (LSAT) is a standardized test used as part of the law school admission process. The LSAT measures skills that are considered essential for success in law school, such as reading comprehension, analytical reasoning, and logical reasoning.

The LSAT is administered four times a year at testing centers around the world. In the year 2022, over 100,000 individuals took the LSAT. The test is a half-day, multiple-choice examination that takes approximately four hours to complete, including a 35-minute writing sample. The LSAT consists of six sections, including one writing sample and five 35-minute multiple-choice sections. Each multiple-choice section contains a combination of logical reasoning, analytical reasoning, and reading comprehension questions.

The LSAT consists of four multiple-choice sections, with a total of 101 to 102 questions. The sections are designed to test a wide range of skills, including reading comprehension, analytical reasoning, and logical reasoning.

1. Reading Comprehension: This section tests the student's ability to understand and analyze written material. The questions require the student to

understand the main idea, tone, and arguments presented in the reading passages.
2. Logical Reasoning: This section tests the student's ability to analyze arguments and identify flaws in reasoning. The questions require the student to identify the premises and conclusions of arguments and evaluate the strength of the reasoning.
3. Analytical Reasoning: This section tests the student's ability to analyze a complex system and draw inferences from it. The questions require the student to understand relationships between elements and use this understanding to make deductions.
4. Writing Sample: This section requires the student to write a well-structured, well-reasoned essay in response to a prompt. The writing sample is not scored, but it is sent to law schools as part of the student's LSAT score report.

Grading Criteria:

The LSAT is scored on a scale of 120 to 180, with a median score of about 152. The score is based on the number of questions answered correctly, and the raw score is converted to the scaled score. The conversion process considers the difficulty of the questions and the performance of all test takers in a particular administration.

I took the advice offered below to improve one's score on the LSAT and I did all of the suggestions but get tutoring. I used the ginger juice memory cocktail and filled four huge practice workbooks, I redid old tests, I checked my wrong answers from exams that I had written earlier, and I retain all materials to this day. I prepped an inordinate amount, by that I mean hundreds of hours for no increase in my score at all.

I feel that the LSAT was biased toward people that had studied statistics and probability as the workbooks often drew bell curves to solve problems. It is not guaranteed that a person will improve each time they take the LSAT, but it is possible if they prepare properly. Preparation is key to improving on the LSAT. Some ways to prepare include:

1. Familiarizing yourself with the test format and types of questions: Understanding the structure of the LSAT and the types of questions it asks can help you feel more confident on test day and make the most of your time.
2. Studying previous LSAT exams: Practicing with previous LSAT exams can give you a better idea of the types of questions you will encounter on the test.
3. Utilizing LSAT prep materials: There are many LSAT prep materials available, including books, study guides, and practice exams. These materials can help you build your skills and confidence in the areas tested by the LSAT.

4. Working with a tutor or taking an LSAT prep course: A tutor or an LSAT prep course can provide personalized feedback and guidance to help you improve your performance.

5. Focusing on your weaknesses: Identifying and addressing your weaknesses is an important part of improving your LSAT score. This may mean spending more time studying certain areas or working with a tutor to improve your skills.

I scored just slightly better than one-half of everyone who wrote the exam. I attempted the exam five times and scored the exact same every time.

As I write this book, a nagging question has been on my mind: should I take an IQ test at the age of 74? It's been said that test scores tend to decline with age, and while I believe I am still operating at about 80% of my former capabilities, it would be foolish to assume my scores haven't been impacted by time. To be honest, I've never even received a straight answer as to what my IQ is.

Back in 1973, when I was just 22 years old, I took an official IQ test and thought I had done quite well. The test administrator had been observing me for two weeks, conducting behavioral tests as well. Before agreeing to take the test, he promised to share my results with me. However, when I finally demanded my score, he seemed to be in competition with me and resentful of my high result. Rather than disclosing my score, he simply said that I was in the top ten percent but claimed that IQ tests were meaningless and that a person's score was simply a matter of speed. In fact, he went as far as to say that timing the dilation of a person's eyeball would be just as accurate as administering an IQ test. Despite my attempts to convince him to honor his promise, I was unable to obtain my actual score.

I think that I am most likely still in the top fifteen percent and may still write an IQ test if I can find a legitimate provider that I can trust. I have gotten halfway through some online testing sites that crashed or offered a chance to resubmit wrong answers. Some will sell you a score of 129 and above for a cash payment.

Intelligence Quotient (IQ) is a score obtained from standardized tests that are designed to measure an individual's cognitive abilities and potential for intellectual development. The concept of IQ was first introduced in the early 20th century and has since become a widely used and often controversial tool for evaluating cognitive abilities.

IQ tests typically measure a range of cognitive skills and abilities, including verbal ability, reasoning, spatial visualization, and memory. The score obtained from an IQ test is intended to provide a measure of an individual's general cognitive abilities relative to others of the same age.

One of the most well-known IQ tests is the Stanford-Binet Intelligence Scale, which was first developed in the early 1900s and has been revised several times over the years. The Stanford-Binet measures a range of abilities, including verbal comprehension, mathematical ability, spatial visualization, and memory.

The concept of IQ has been the subject of much debate among psychologists and other experts. One of the main criticisms of IQ tests is that they may not accurately reflect an individual's true cognitive abilities and potential. IQ tests can be affected by a range of factors, including cultural and socioeconomic background, language, and prior education.

Another criticism of IQ tests is that they may reflect only a narrow range of cognitive abilities and may not accurately measure other important qualities, such as creativity, emotional intelligence, or practical intelligence. It is important to note that IQ tests are not the only measure of intelligence, and there are other ways of evaluating an individual's cognitive abilities and potential for intellectual development.

IQ scores are typically reported as a single number that represents an individual's relative cognitive abilities compared to others of the same age. The average IQ score is 100, with a standard deviation of 15. This means that approximately 68% of the population has an IQ score between 85 and 115. Here are some common classifications of IQ scores:

1. Above average: IQ scores of 115 or above are considered above average. A score of 130 or above is considered in the top 2% of the population.
2. Average: An IQ score of 100 is considered average. The majority of the population falls into this category, with scores ranging from 85 to 115.
3. Below average: IQ scores below 85 are considered below average. A score of 70 or below is considered in the bottom 2% of the population.
4. Gifted: A score of 130 or above is often considered the threshold for giftedness. Individuals with a score in this range are considered to have exceptional cognitive abilities and may require special education and support to reach their full potential.
5. Intellectual disability: A score of 70 or below is often considered the threshold for intellectual disability. Individuals with this classification may require special education and support to learn basic life skills and function independently.

It is important to note that IQ scores are only one measure of cognitive abilities and should not be used as the sole determinant of an individual's potential for intellectual development. IQ scores should also be considered in conjunction with other factors, such as education, cultural background, and socioeconomic status. Additionally, IQ scores can change over time, and may not accurately reflect an individual's true cognitive abilities at all times.

I have an enquiring mind and I have always been an avid reader. In the early 80's while living in Vancouver I found a copy of Rapaport Gill and Schafer's *Diagnostic Psychological Testing*. I read it and try as I may I cannot forget it. So, the question has arisen as to whether or not this made me a 'cheater' on subsequent exams. Here is what happened to me.

The examiner asked me the question that earlier I had not known the answer to. Who wrote Faust? This one question moves someone from having a post-secondary education such as a grade twelve high school diploma to being equivalent to having a university degree. (something that I badly wanted but at the time had not achieved) I did not cheat and although I knew the answer, I also knew it was on the test, so I merely repeated the question Faust? As if I had never heard of Faust before. "Faust" is a German legend that was popularized in the 19th century by the German author Johann Wolfgang von Goethe. He wrote a two-part play titled "Faust Part One" and "Faust Part Two," which tells the story of a man named Faust who makes a deal with the devil, Mephistopheles, exchanging his soul for unlimited knowledge and worldly pleasures.

Goethe's "Faust" is considered a masterpiece of German literature and is one of the most famous works in the German language. It explores themes of redemption, the human condition, and the dangers of unchecked ambition and desire. The play has been adapted into various forms of media, including plays, operas, and films, and continues to be widely read and studied today.

I undid this honorable action a few minutes later when he accusatorily said that I should admit to having read books on diagnostic testing. Because I was feeling like I had been caught cheating I denied it. I really never lie. I always tell the truth because to my way of thinking; that lying is because someone is afraid of the truth, and I never want to be afraid of the truth.

I take the concept of truth to extremes. Like not wanting to swear upon a bible "so help me god" as I do not truly believe in these things. I would rather affirm. When I got my government Security Clearance I had to take an Oath of Secrecy and an Oath of Allegiance to the Crown. This was problematic because I had some questions as to if Canada needed a foreign sovereign. My point is that we aspies agonize over moral questions that seem trifling to normal people.

We have a naïve belief in social justice and we seem to discount lying because we never do it ourselves.

While we really lack empathy for the victims, we want to restore order to the system with fair trials. We are constantly shocked when we see people lie to get themselves out of legal difficulties.

Not getting jokes and not knowing when someone is pulling your leg is embarrassing for people like me with ASD. People with ASD may experience difficulties understanding sarcasm due to our tendency to interpret language literally. This can lead to misunderstandings and misinterpretations, particularly in social situations where sarcasm is often used as a tool for conveying humor or expressing emotions indirectly.

People with ASD may have trouble recognizing and interpreting social cues such as facial expressions, tone of voice, and body language, which are essential in understanding the intended meaning behind sarcasm. Additionally, individuals with ASD often think in concrete and literal terms, making it difficult for them to grasp abstract concepts like sarcasm. These challenges with recognizing and understanding sarcasm can have a significant impact on social interaction and communication for individuals with ASD.

Not appreciating social boundaries draws attention to people like me with ASD I kept writing and failing the LSAT and would just not give up. That was to study law out of general interest as I had no intentions of ever practicing law.

My interest in law is also puzzling. I know in my heart that some judge would have me disbarred before too long. I am merely interested in how just decisions are made in court. I study procedures and court rules in great detail.

I have won several large and significant cases. I have argued against the likes of Faskin Martineau and won. Fasken is a leading international law firm with a reputation for delivering exceptional legal services. With roots dating back over 150 years, the firm has grown to become one of the largest full-service law firms in Canada, with offices in Toronto, Vancouver, Montréal, Ottawa, London, and Johannesburg.

In terms of influence, Fasken is widely regarded as one of the leading law firms in Canada and is highly respected by clients, competitors, and legal industry commentators. The firm has a strong track record of delivering successful outcomes for clients and has a reputation for being one of the most dynamic and innovative law firms in the country.

My company sued Cummins in Edmonton Alberta and the case dragged on for years. Their defense was always brilliant, and their lawyers put up a solid defense. I used young lawyers just starting out at a firm that did more divorces than commercial litigation. In all five or six lawyers had to be introduced to the complicated warranty case and brought up to speed on my strategies. I won that case in a David verses Goliath epic legal battle that I thoroughly enjoyed.

On the criminal side of the law, I was successful in defending my house from seizure by the court three times in three estreatment hearings where my house was to be seized by the Manitoba court system. A native woman whom I had bailed out was charged with violating bail conditions by moving without informing the court. But we had informed the court of the change of address. Then they claimed that she had missed court and used a returned envelope from the old address as evidence that she had been notified of the appearance date.

I think it was a warning to me that I should stop giving legal advice to native women who were trying to stop the government from seizing their newborn children. I was banned from the courtroom for the sake of the privacy of the baby that was being apprehended. I had tried claiming that I was acting as a legal interpreter because they were natives but that was also disallowed.

I sound like a grievance collector, but I am trying to demonstrate my quixotic nature. I feel that my generation did achieve our two main goals. We stopped the war in Vietnam and got cannabis legalized.

"Neuroplasticity: The Brain that Heals Itself" by Norman Doidge is a comprehensive and well-researched book that explores the concept of neuroplasticity and its impact on the human brain. The author provides a detailed and engaging account of how the brain can change and adapt throughout our lives, and how this has far-reaching implications for our health and well-being.

One of the strengths of this book is its accessibility. The author presents complex scientific concepts in a way that is easy to understand and provides a range of case studies and examples to illustrate how neuroplasticity works in practice. The book also covers a wide range of topics, from brain development in childhood to the effects of injury and disease on the brain and provides a wealth of information on how we can harness neuroplasticity to improve our lives.

One of the standout aspects of the book is its discussion of the potential of neuroplasticity in helping to heal the brain after injury or disease. The author provides evidence of how neuroplastic changes in the brain can help to rewire and recover lost functions and provides inspiring examples of individuals who have used neuroplasticity to recover from conditions such as stroke, traumatic brain injury, and chronic pain.

Another strength of the book is its discussion of the implications of neuroplasticity for the way we think about brain development and aging. The author argues that neuroplasticity gives us the power to reshape our own brains and provides evidence of how we can use this power to prevent or delay the effects of aging on the brain.

Neuroplasticity refers to the ability of the brain to change and reorganize itself in response to new experiences and environmental stimuli. This capacity for change is what enables the brain to recover from injury, adapt to new situations, and learn new skills. Neuroplasticity is a critical aspect of brain function and has been the subject of much research in recent years, particularly in the field of rehabilitation medicine.

One of the most well-known examples of neuroplasticity is the brain's ability to recover from injury. After a stroke, for example, the brain can rewire itself to compensate for the damaged areas, allowing the individual to recover some or all of their lost abilities. This process is known as neuroplasticity-mediated recovery, and it occurs through the formation of new neural connections in undamaged parts of the brain. With proper rehabilitation, individuals with stroke-related impairments can often regain some of their lost abilities, such as movement, speech, and sensory perception.

Another example of neuroplasticity is seen in the process of learning new skills. When a person learns a new task, such as playing a musical instrument or speaking a new language, their brain reorganizes itself to support this new skill. This process occurs through the formation of new neural connections and the strengthening of existing connections, and it allows the individual to become more proficient in the new skill over time.

Clinical studies have demonstrated the effectiveness of neuroplasticity-based interventions in improving outcomes for individuals with a range of neurological conditions. For example, studies have shown that patients with Parkinson's disease who undergo intensive physical therapy can improve their motor skills and reduce their symptoms. Similarly, studies have found that individuals with chronic pain can experience significant reductions in pain levels through the use of neuroplasticity-based interventions, such as mindfulness-based meditation and cognitive-behavioral therapy.

In addition to these examples, neuroplasticity has also been shown to play a role in the development and treatment of mental health conditions, such as depression and anxiety. For example, studies have found that individuals with depression who participate in physical exercise or mindfulness-based meditation can experience improvements in their symptoms, likely due to changes in the brain's structure and function. The brain's ability to change in response to these interventions is thought to be related to changes in neurotransmitter levels and increased activity in specific regions of the brain.

In the field of rehabilitation medicine, neuroplasticity-based interventions are often used in combination with other treatments, such as physical therapy, to maximize their effectiveness. For example, patients with spinal cord injury may receive physical therapy to improve their mobility and dexterity, along with cognitive-behavioral therapy to manage their pain and improve their quality of life. Similarly, patients with traumatic brain injury may receive physical therapy to improve their motor function and cognitive-behavioral therapy to manage their symptoms, such as memory loss, headaches, and mood changes.

Chapter 12: Diagnosis Demystified: The Process of Standard Diagnostic Testing for ASD

The Wechsler-Bellevue Intelligence Scale is a widely used tool for measuring cognitive abilities and intellectual functioning. Developed by David Wechsler in 1939, the Wechsler-Bellevue scale is a comprehensive evaluation tool that measures various aspects of cognitive function, including verbal and nonverbal reasoning, memory, and problem-solving abilities. Over the years, the scale has been revised and updated to reflect advances in our understanding of human cognition and to ensure its continued relevance and usefulness.

The Wechsler-Bellevue scale consists of a series of subtests that are designed to measure different aspects of cognitive function. These subtests include verbal and nonverbal tasks, such as vocabulary, arithmetic, and picture completion, as well as more complex tasks that assess reasoning, memory, and problem-solving abilities. The subtests are designed to be both engaging and challenging, and they are administered in a standardized manner to ensure accurate and consistent results.

One of the key features of the Wechsler-Bellevue scale is its focus on measuring both verbal and nonverbal abilities. This approach is based on the idea that intelligence is not a single, unitary construct, but rather a complex combination of different cognitive abilities that can vary independently of one another. By measuring both verbal and nonverbal abilities, the Wechsler-Bellevue scale provides a more comprehensive and nuanced understanding of an individual's intellectual functioning.

The Wechsler-Bellevue scale is used in a variety of settings, including clinical, educational, and research settings. In clinical settings, the scale is often used to evaluate individuals with suspected cognitive impairments or learning disabilities, as well as individuals with developmental disorders, such as autism spectrum disorder. The scale can also be used to evaluate individuals with neurological conditions, such as brain injury or dementia, or those with mental health conditions, such as depression or anxiety.

In educational settings, the Wechsler-Bellevue scale is often used to evaluate the intellectual abilities of children and adolescents. This information can be used to determine eligibility for special education services, to identify areas of strength and weakness, and to inform educational planning. In research settings, the Wechsler-Bellevue scale is often used as a measure of cognitive ability in studies investigating brain-behavior relationships, as well as in studies examining the development and aging of the brain.

One of the strengths of the Wechsler-Bellevue scale is its well-established validity and reliability. The scale has been extensively tested and validated in a wide range of populations and is widely recognized as a reliable and valid measure of cognitive abilities. Additionally, the scale is regularly updated to reflect advances in our understanding of human cognition and to ensure its continued relevance and usefulness.

Another strength of the Wechsler-Bellevue scale is its versatility. The scale can be used to evaluate individuals across the lifespan, from early childhood through adulthood, and it can be adapted to meet the needs of different populations, such as individuals with developmental disabilities or neurological conditions. The scale is also available in multiple languages, making it accessible to individuals from diverse backgrounds

The Babcock Story Recall Test is a measure of verbal memory and learning, designed to assess an individual's ability to recall and retain information over a short period of time. The test was developed by psychologist George Babcock in the early 1900s and remains a widely used tool in the assessment of memory and learning abilities.

The Babcock Story Recall Test involves the presentation of a short narrative or story, typically consisting of several sentences or paragraphs, to the individual being tested. The individual is then asked to recall as much of the story as they can, either immediately after hearing it or after a short delay. The recall can be either free recall, where the individual is free to recall the story in any order they choose, or serial recall, where the individual is asked to recall the story in the same order as it was presented.

The Babcock Story Recall Test is typically used in clinical, educational, and research settings to assess an individual's ability to encode, store, and retrieve information from memory. The test can provide valuable information about an individual's memory function, including their capacity to hold information in short-term memory, their ability to organize and integrate information, and their ability to recall information over time.

In clinical settings, the Babcock Story Recall Test is often used to assess individuals with suspected cognitive impairments, such as those with neurological conditions, mental health conditions, or learning disabilities. The test can help to identify specific memory deficits and to inform treatment planning and intervention strategies.

In educational settings, the Babcock Story Recall Test is often used to assess the memory abilities of children and adolescents. This information can be used to identify areas of strength and weakness and to inform educational planning and support.

In research settings, the Babcock Story Recall Test is often used as a measure of verbal memory in studies investigating the relationship between memory and other cognitive abilities, as well as in studies examining the effects of aging and disease on memory function.

Word association tests are scored based on the time it takes an individual to respond to a stimulus word with a related word. The response time, along with the content of the response, are used to determine an individual's score.

In a word association test, the individual is presented with a stimulus word and asked to provide the first word that comes to mind in response. The response time is recorded and used as a measure of the individual's ability to access and retrieve information from memory. Shorter response times are typically seen as an indication of greater fluency and faster information processing, while longer response times may indicate slower processing or a difficulty accessing information from memory.

The content of the response is also taken into account when scoring a word association test. The response is evaluated for its relevance and relatedness to the stimulus word, with responses that are more closely related to the stimulus word typically seen as more favorable. Responses that are unrelated or tangential to the stimulus word may indicate a difficulty in accessing relevant information or a lack of association between the stimulus word and related words.

In addition to the time and content of the response, the consistency of the individual's responses is also taken into account. Responses that are consistent across trials and are closely related to the stimulus words are seen as more favorable and may indicate greater fluency and better organization of information in memory.

Overall, the score on a word association test is a composite of the time it takes to respond, the content of the response, and the consistency of the response. This information is used to provide insight into an individual's memory and information processing abilities, as well as to identify areas of strength and weakness.

It is important to note that word association tests are not diagnostic tests and should not be used as the sole basis for making clinical decisions. Instead, they are best used as part of a comprehensive evaluation, along with other measures of cognitive functioning, to provide a comprehensive picture of an individual's abilities.

The Rorschach test, also known as the Rorschach inkblot test, is a projective test used in the field of psychology to assess an individual's personality and emotional functioning. The test is administered by presenting an individual with a series of ten standardized inkblots and asking them to describe what they see in each image.

In the Rorschach test, the responses given by an individual to the inkblots are thought to reveal their underlying personality traits, attitudes, and emotions. The responses are evaluated based on a number of factors, including the content of the response, the number of elements described in the image, the type of response (e.g., is it a complete or fragmentary response), and the perceived emotion or attitude conveyed by the response.

The Rorschach test is used in diagnosis to assess a wide range of psychological disorders and conditions, including depression, anxiety, psychotic disorders, personality disorders, and thought disorders. The test is thought to provide insight into an individual's unconscious thoughts, emotions, and motivations, which can help to inform the diagnosis and treatment of various mental health conditions.

However, it is important to note that the use of the Rorschach test in diagnosis is controversial, and there is ongoing debate about its reliability and validity. Some researchers and clinicians question the accuracy and usefulness of the test, and there is a lack of empirical evidence to support its use in many cases.

As such, the Rorschach test should not be used as the sole basis for making a diagnosis. Instead, it is best used as part of a comprehensive evaluation, along with other measures of psychological functioning, to provide a more complete picture of an individual's mental health and functioning. Additionally, it is important that the test be administered and interpreted by a trained and experienced professional, as the results can be highly influenced by the individual administering the test.

The Thematic Apperception Test (TAT) is a projective test used in the field of psychology to assess an individual's personality, emotional functioning, and motivations. The test is administered by presenting an individual with a series of standardized picture stimuli and asking them to create a story about each picture. The stories created by the individual are then used to provide insight into their unconscious thoughts, emotions, and motivations.

The TAT was first developed in the 1930s by Henry Murray and Christiana Morgan and has since become a widely used tool in the assessment of personality and emotional functioning. The test consists of a set of 31 standardized cards, each of which depicts an ambiguous scene or image, such as a person looking out a window or a group of people in a room.

The individual being tested is asked to create a story about each picture, including information about the characters, their motivations and emotions, and what is happening in the scene. The responses are then evaluated based on a number of factors, including the content of the response, the type of response (e.g., is it a complete or fragmentary response), the perceived emotion or attitude conveyed by the response, and the individual's use of defensive mechanisms such as repression or denial.

The TAT is thought to provide insight into an individual's unconscious thoughts, emotions, and motivations. It is used to assess a wide range of psychological disorders and conditions, including depression, anxiety, personality disorders, and thought disorders. The test is also used to evaluate an individual's emotional and interpersonal functioning, including their capacity for empathy and their ability to form healthy relationships.

However, it is important to note that the use of the TAT in diagnosis is controversial, and there is ongoing debate about its reliability and validity. Some researchers and clinicians question the accuracy and usefulness of the test, and there is a lack of empirical evidence to support its use in many cases.

As such, the TAT should not be used as the sole basis for making a diagnosis. Instead, it is best used as part of a comprehensive evaluation, along with other measures of psychological functioning, to provide a more complete picture of an individual's mental health and functioning. Additionally, it is important that the test be administered and interpreted by a trained and experienced professional, as the results can be highly influenced by the individual administering the test.

Scatter in psychological testing refers to the variability in scores that a person may receive across different tests. It represents the range of scores a person may receive, from the highest score to the lowest score, on a series of tests. In other words, scatter represents the spread of scores in a person's test results.

For example, if a person takes several tests to assess their cognitive ability, and receives scores of 100, 95, 90, and 85, the scatter of their scores would be 100-85=15. This indicates that the person's scores vary by 15 points across the different tests.

Scatter in a person's test scores can be seen as a measure of their consistency in performance. High scatter indicates that a person's scores are more inconsistent, while low scatter suggests that their scores are more consistent. A person with high scatter in their test scores may perform well on one test but poorly on another, whereas a person with low scatter may consistently score around the same range.

Scatter in test scores can also provide valuable information about a person's strengths and weaknesses. For example, if a person consistently scores high on tests of verbal ability but low on tests of numerical ability, this may indicate that they have a strength in language-related skills and a weakness in mathematical skills.

Scatter in test scores can be influenced by a variety of factors, such as test-taking anxiety, fatigue, attentional problems, or simply the nature of the test. When scatter is high, it can be difficult to interpret the results of psychological tests and make accurate assessments. On the other hand, low scatter in test scores can indicate that the results are more reliable and consistent, making them easier to interpret and use in making assessments.

A state-of-the-art semi truck simulator training system is designed to provide an immersive and realistic experience for trainees. It typically consists of a cockpit or cab that closely resembles the interior of a real semi truck, including the steering wheel, pedals, and other controls. The cockpit provides a physically and visually convincing simulation environment that allows the trainee to practice driving and handling the truck in a safe and controlled setting.

The visual display system is a key component of the simulator, providing a realistic representation of the road and surrounding environment. The display typically includes large, high-resolution screens that provide an expansive field of view, as well as specialized graphics hardware and software that deliver realistic lighting, shadows, and other visual effects. In some cases, the display system may also include motion sensing or motion tracking technology that provides a more immersive experience by allowing the trainee to feel the motion of the vehicle.

To further enhance the realism of the simulation, the state-of-the-art semi truck simulator training system may also incorporate a wide range of sensors and other hardware that can replicate the behavior of a real truck. For example, it may include sensors that simulate the resistance of the steering wheel and pedals, as well as systems that generate vibrations, sounds, and other sensory cues that are associated with driving a truck.

In addition to providing a realistic simulation environment, the state-of-the-art semi truck simulator training system may also include advanced training software and analytical tools that allow trainers to assess the performance of the trainees, track their progress, and provide customized feedback. This can help to ensure that trainees are fully prepared to operate a semi truck when they are ready to hit the road.

In a state-of-the-art semi truck simulator training system, sudden snow whiteouts and unexpected obstacles such as pedestrians or dogs running in front of the truck can be simulated to challenge the trainee's decision-making skills and reactions. This is achieved by incorporating advanced software that generates dynamic scenarios, replicating unexpected events that may occur while driving.

During the simulation, the software generates a visual representation of the sudden snow whiteout or obstacle on the display system, and the trainee must respond appropriately. The trainee's actions are recorded and analyzed by the software, and the trainee is provided with feedback on their performance. For example, the software may rate the trainee's speed and distance control, decision-making, and other factors, and provide guidance on how to improve their skills.

By incorporating these dynamic scenarios, the state-of-the-art semi truck simulator training system provides a more realistic and challenging training experience, helping to prepare trainees for real-world scenarios that they may encounter on the road. Additionally, by allowing the trainee to experience these events in a safe and controlled environment, the simulator reduces the risk of accidents or incidents during the training process.

After my commercial truck driver licence had been suspended for medical reasons for two and a half years I got it back. To his credit Dr. Pacin accepted my argument that a provincial driving examiner from the department of motor vehicles should be the one to decide if I was able to safely drive a semi on crowded public highways. I passed the driving exam and my licence was reinstated.

My company Bison Transport accepted me back and put me through a mini orientation and issued me a truck to drive. As I was about to leave the meeting a safety officer from the company said that I had to do some tests on the state of the art simulator. I had been in the simulator before and I did not like it.

To me everything happening in the simulator is real. If they make one of my steer tires blow out speeding downhill around corners, I think that I am about to rollover. If they make me hit a car or a dog I think that it really happened for a second.

I was angry at having to take the test and I hated the machine. I did not like the guy who was conducting the test but I felt that I would just plow through it and get back to work. The tester threw every hazard in the book at me. Dogs running out in front of me, cars swerving into my lane, sudden whiteout blizzard conditions, and jackknife scenarios.

I was relieved to be done and he came around with some computer printouts scratching his head and apologizing. I would have to repeat the test because the simulation must have been out of calibration. So reluctantly I did the ten-minute test again. I was angry and my adrenalin was pumping hard. I resolved to pass the test this time and I did everything at full speed.

He came around to the door of the simulator with an air of victory. He waved the printouts enthusiastically and praised me with genuine astonishment. He told me that I had done it twice and the results were the same proving that the machine had not been out of calibration.

I knew how long Bison had had the simulator. In about three years the simulator had tested thousands of truckers. Excitedly he waved the printouts under my nose exclaiming that my speed was orders of magnitude faster than anyone had ever been. "Beyond Off the Chart" as I think he put it. I angrily asked what he would be saying if I had been the slowest. That he had lied to me when he said it did not matter how I did, and that it was not being recorded on my driver file.

I know that this is not a scientific test, and I cannot prove that he was not lying to me or that in fact the simulator really was making an error. I have always felt that I am extremely fast, and this seems like confirmation.

I have always tried to study other people in timed situations trying to get a handle on what is above average reflexes. I think a simple pupil dilation test could time my speed as well as anything. I watch drag racing to see people with extremely fast reaction time. Hocky goalies, quick-fire competitive shooting sports,

Formula One drivers, and 100-meter Olympic sprinters fascinate me with their reaction times.

I have a home gym and I especially like to use my boxing speed bag. Some people call it a rhythm bag. I train on it for speed and go so fast that the only way to tell how things are going is by the sound. The bag is a blur. I set up combos and do rhythm drills that sound good. I see many boxers use the back of their hands on a speed bag, but I do not do that. I use proper overhand punches which is much more difficult to do fast.

The "Christmas Tree" in Top Fueler NHRA drag racing consists of a series of vertically mounted lights that signal the start of the race. These lights include:

- The yellow lights: There are three yellow lights that illuminate in succession, counting down to the start of the race. The yellow lights serve as a warning to the drivers to prepare for the start.
- The red light: The red light illuminates when the race is about to begin. If a driver engages the throttle before the red light goes off, it is called a "red light violation," and they are disqualified from the race.
- The green light: The green light signals the start of the race. When the green light goes on, the drivers engage the throttle and race down the track.

The Christmas Tree is designed to provide a fair and accurate starting signal to the drivers, and the reaction time to the green light is a critical factor in determining the outcome of the race. Top Fueler drivers must have quick reflexes and be able to accurately react to the lights in order to achieve the best off-the-line speed and get a head start on their competition.

In Top Fuel, Cory McClenathan has an average reaction time of 0.089, followed by Larry Dixon with 0.070. In Funny Car, Tony Pedregon has the fastest average reaction time of 0.073, followed by John Force with 0.085, and Ashley Force Hood with 0.115. In Pro Stock, Greg Stanfield has the fastest average reaction time of 0.024, followed by Rickie Jones with 0.022, and Mike Edwards with 0.043.

Bob Munden held 18 Guinness Book records for doing this shooting drill. He drew and fired a Colt single-action revolver in less than 2 tenths of a second. Moments later, after the loading of the gun by an official observer to actually prove that it contained 2 cartridges, he drew and fired that same pistol twice in exactly .2 seconds.

Reflex times are the duration between a stimulus and the resulting response. In motor sports, particularly Formula One, drivers need to have fast reflex times in order to react quickly to changing conditions and make split-second decisions. These decisions and reactions occur at high speeds, and even a small delay can result in a loss of control or an accident.

The average human reflex time is around 250 milliseconds. However, top athletes and professionals in high-stress situations, such as F1 drivers, often have reflex times that are significantly faster than average. These faster reflex times are the result of both innate ability and extensive training.

In Formula One auto racing, drivers train to improve their reflex times through various methods, such as reaction-time drills, physical and mental conditioning, and simulation exercises. By improving their reflex times, F1 drivers are better equipped to make quick decisions, respond to changing conditions, and maintain control of their car at high speeds.

The fast reflexes of National Hockey League (NHL) goalies are a critical component of their success on the ice. Goalies need to react quickly to incoming shots, which can approach 100 mph, and make split-second decisions on how to make the save.

To put this into perspective, research has shown that the average reaction time for an NHL goalie is around 0.2 to 0.3 seconds. However, elite NHL goalies have been recorded to have reaction times as low as 0.1 seconds, allowing them to make saves that appear to be miraculous.

One example of a top NHL goalie with lightning-fast reflexes is Carey Price of the Montreal Canadiens. He is known for his quick reactions and ability to make game-changing saves. In a game against the Toronto Maple Leafs, Price made a save on a shot from close range that was clocked at 102 mph. Despite the speed of the shot, Price was able to react quickly and make the save, preserving the lead for his team.

Another example is Andrei Vasilevskiy of the Tampa Bay Lightning. Vasilevskiy has consistently been one of the top goalies in the NHL, and his reflexes play a major role in his success. In a game against the Detroit Red Wings, Vasilevskiy made a save on a shot that was taken from just outside the crease. The shot was clocked at over 100 mph, but Vasilevskiy was able to react quickly and catch the puck in his glove.

Overall, the fast reflexes of NHL goalies are a crucial aspect of their performance and a key factor in their ability to make game-changing saves. These reflexes are the result of a combination of innate ability and years of training and practice.

In the Olympic 100-meter race, athletes' reflexes play a crucial role in their performance, particularly at the start of the race. A sprinter's reaction time, or the time it takes for them to respond to the starting gun, can be the difference between a good start and a slow start, which can greatly impact the outcome of the race.

The average reaction time for sprinters in the 100-meter race is around 0.165 seconds. However, elite sprinters have been recorded to have reaction times as low as 0.100 seconds, which can give them a significant advantage at the start of the race.

For example, Usain Bolt, who is considered one of the greatest sprinters of all time, had an average reaction time of 0.155 seconds in his prime. This allowed him to get out of the blocks quickly and establish an early lead, which he was then able to maintain through the rest of the race.

Another example is Tyson Gay, who was known for his quick reaction time and explosive start. Gay's reaction time was clocked at 0.128 seconds in a race, which allowed him to get out of the blocks quickly and establish an early lead.

The best clinical test for reaction time varies based on the purpose of the measurement and the population being tested. A simple reaction time test measures the time it takes for a person to respond to a single visual or auditory stimulus and is a basic measure of reaction time. However, more complex tests can be used to measure more specific aspects of reaction time, such as choice reaction time (the time it takes for a person to choose between two or more stimuli) or multiple-choice reaction time (the time it takes for a person to choose between many stimuli).

In addition to these basic measures, there are also tests that measure reaction time in specific contexts, such as reaction time while performing a task, or reaction time under different conditions, such as while tired or stressed. The best test to use depends on the purpose of the measurement and the specific factors that are being evaluated.

The minimum human reaction time varies depending on several factors, such as age, fatigue, stress, and the type of reaction being measured (e.g., simple reaction time, choice reaction time). However, on average, a simple reaction time for an adult is typically around 200-250 milliseconds. This means that it takes an adult about 200-250 milliseconds to respond to a simple, sudden stimulus, such as a visual or auditory cue.

Choice reaction time, which involves the selection of a response from multiple options, is typically slower than simple reaction time, with average values ranging from 300-500 milliseconds or more.

It is important to note that these are average values, and that individual variability can be substantial. Additionally, factors such as age, fatigue, and stress can affect reaction time and may result in longer or shorter reaction times for a given individual.

Suzanne Somers is a familiar name to many due to her prominent role in the hit television series 'Three's Company' and other acting gigs. During an interview about her son's health, she described symptoms that closely resembled what I had been experiencing with increasing frequency.

These symptoms included excessive sweating on my face, low levels of testosterone, a persistent feeling of fatigue, and bulbar effect, all of which started after I suffered a head injury resulting in a TBI. The Bulbar effect, also known as pseudobulbar palsy, is a medical condition characterized by difficulty in controlling the muscles responsible for speech, swallowing, and facial expressions. The condition is usually caused by damage to the lower motor neurons in the brainstem or cranial nerves, resulting in the loss of voluntary control over these muscles.

Individuals with the Bulbar effect may experience symptoms such as slurred speech, nasal speech, difficulty in swallowing food and liquids, choking or coughing while eating or drinking, drooling, and involuntary facial expressions. These symptoms can be severe, making communication and eating difficult and uncomfortable for the affected person.

The condition can be caused by several factors, including neurodegenerative diseases such as amyotrophic lateral sclerosis (ALS), multiple sclerosis,

Parkinson's disease, traumatic brain injury, stroke, and certain infections.

The treatment of the Bulbar effect depends on the underlying cause and severity of the symptoms. For instance, individuals with mild symptoms may benefit from speech therapy, whereas those with severe symptoms may require a feeding tube or other supportive devices to help with eating and drinking. Additionally, medications such as muscle relaxants or anti-spasmodic agents may be prescribed to alleviate symptoms. In severe cases, surgery may be necessary to relieve pressure on the cranial nerves.

In addition to the symptoms mentioned earlier, spontaneous crying or laughing is also a common feature of the Bulbar effect. This symptom is known as emotional lability, and it occurs due to the loss of control over the facial muscles responsible for expressing emotions. As a result, individuals with this condition may experience sudden and uncontrollable outbursts of laughter or crying, often at inappropriate times. I would be talking to someone and not realize that tears were flowing down my cheeks. I had occasional sudden crying episodes for no apparent reason while I was not at all sad or upset.

Based on my symptoms, I suspected that I might have an adenoma of my pituitary gland, a small grape-sized organ situated directly behind the eyes and under the brain. If left untreated, an adenoma could grow and compress the optic nerve, leading to blindness. My endocrinologist was very surprised when an MRI proved my self-diagnosis to be correct. I had a 7-millimetre adenoma of the pituitary. He referred me to a neurosurgeon for treatment. Surgery would occur once the size grew to 10 mm.

The pituitary gland, also known as the hypophysis, is a small endocrine gland located at the base of the brain. It is considered the "master gland" due to its crucial role in regulating various physiological processes through the release of hormones.

The pituitary gland is divided into two main sections: the anterior pituitary (or adenohypophysis) and the posterior pituitary (or neurohypophysis). The anterior pituitary secretes hormones that regulate growth (growth hormone), reproduction (follicle-stimulating hormone and luteinizing hormone), and metabolism (thyroid-stimulating hormone and adrenocorticotropic hormone). The posterior pituitary, on the other hand, stores, and releases two hormones produced by nerve cells in the hypothalamus: antidiuretic hormone (ADH), which regulates water balance in the body, and oxytocin, which plays a role in reproduction and maternal behavior.

Dysfunction of the pituitary gland can result in a variety of medical conditions. For example, if the anterior pituitary gland fails to produce enough hormones, it can result in growth hormone deficiency (dwarfism), hypogonadism, or adrenal insufficiency. Conversely, an overproduction of hormones from the anterior pituitary can result in conditions such as acromegaly (excessive growth), gigantism (excessive growth in children), or Cushing's disease.

Damage to the pituitary gland can also result from injury, tumor growth, or radiation therapy, leading to decreased hormone production and function. Treatment for pituitary gland disorders typically involves hormone replacement therapy, surgical removal of tumors, or radiation therapy.

A 7mm adenoma of the pituitary is a benign (non-cancerous) growth on the pituitary gland, which is located at the base of the brain and controls the release of hormones that regulate important bodily functions such as growth, metabolism, and reproductive processes.

A 7mm size adenoma is considered small but can still have significant impact on the function of the pituitary gland. The diagnosis of a 7mm pituitary adenoma is typically made through imaging tests such as MRI or CT scans.

The clinical assessment of a 7mm pituitary adenoma would involve evaluating the patient's symptoms, medical history, and hormonal levels to determine the extent to which the adenoma is affecting the normal functioning of the pituitary gland and overall health. Some common symptoms of pituitary adenomas include headaches, vision changes, fatigue, and changes in menstrual cycles.

If the adenoma is causing hormonal imbalances, the patient may undergo further testing to measure levels of hormones in the blood and determine the type of adenoma present. This information can help determine the most appropriate treatment plan, which may include medication, surgery, or radiation therapy.

It is important to monitor the growth of the adenoma and re-evaluate its impact on the pituitary gland and the patient's overall health, as some pituitary adenomas can grow over time and cause more significant health problems. Regular check-ups with an endocrinologist or neurosurgeon, along with imaging studies and hormone level tests, can help monitor the adenoma and ensure that appropriate treatment is given if needed.

Non-surgical treatments for pituitary adenomas are focused on managing symptoms and regulating hormone imbalances caused by the adenoma. This can be done through medications, such as dopamine agonists, somatostatin analogues, or growth hormone receptor antagonists, which can help reduce the size of the adenoma and control hormonal production. In some cases, radiation therapy may also be recommended, where high-energy X-rays are used to destroy the tumor cells and shrink the adenoma.

Another option is called "medical management", which involves close monitoring of hormone levels and regular check-ups to ensure the adenoma is not growing or causing any harm to the body. The type of treatment a patient receives will depend on the specific symptoms and the size and location of the adenoma.

Surgical treatment for pituitary adenomas is often recommended when the adenoma is large, causing significant symptoms, or is resistant to medical treatments. The goal of surgery is to remove as much of the adenoma as possible, while preserving normal pituitary function. The most common surgical procedure for pituitary adenomas is transsphenoidal surgery. This involves accessing the pituitary gland through the nose, rather than through a large incision on the skull, minimizing damage to surrounding healthy tissues. The procedure is performed under general anesthesia and involves removal of the adenoma through the sphenoid sinus. In some cases, where the adenoma is very large or has invaded surrounding tissues, a craniotomy may be necessary, which involves removing a portion of the skull to access the adenoma. After surgery, the patient will be monitored for hormone levels and other symptoms to ensure the adenoma has been fully removed and the pituitary gland is functioning normally.

Medications can play a role in managing pituitary adenomas by reducing symptoms and slowing down tumor growth. The specific type of medication used will depend on the type of hormone that the adenoma is producing.

Dopamine agonists are commonly used to treat prolactinomas, which are adenomas that produce too much prolactin, a hormone involved in milk production. These medications mimic the effects of dopamine, a hormone that normally regulates prolactin secretion. They can lower prolactin levels, shrink the tumor, and alleviate symptoms such as breast tenderness and milk production in women, or impotence and decreased sex drive in men.

Somatostatin analogs, such as octreotide, are used to treat growth hormone-secreting adenomas. These medications mimic somatostatin, a hormone that regulates growth hormone secretion. They can reduce the secretion of growth hormone and, as a result, shrink the tumor and improve symptoms such as acromegaly (excessive growth of bones, particularly in the face, hands, and feet) and diabetes.

Cabergoline and bromocriptine are medications that can be used to lower prolactin levels and shrink prolactinomas. They work by blocking the secretion of prolactin and reducing the size of the tumor. In some cases, medications may be used in combination with surgery or radiation therapy. The goal of these treatments is to manage symptoms and control the growth of the adenoma while minimizing side effects.

It's important to work with a doctor to find the best treatment plan for your individual situation.

Charlotte's Web CBD is a hemp-derived cannabidiol (CBD) product that is marketed for various health benefits, including reducing seizures and improving symptoms of autism spectrum disorder (ASD). However, it is important to note that the evidence for the efficacy of Charlotte's Web CBD for these conditions is limited and more research is needed to confirm its effectiveness.

CBD has been shown in some studies to have anticonvulsant properties, which may be beneficial for reducing the frequency and severity of seizures. This has led to the use of CBD-based products, including Charlotte's Web CBD, as a treatment option for people with epilepsy, particularly those with treatment-resistant epilepsy. However, more well-designed clinical trials are needed to determine the safety and efficacy of Charlotte's Web CBD for this condition.

As for the effects of Charlotte's Web CBD on ASD, the current evidence is limited, and more research is needed. Some studies have suggested that CBD may improve symptoms such as anxiety, sleep problems, and irritability in people with ASD. However, the results of these studies are mixed and further research is needed to confirm the safety and efficacy of Charlotte's Web CBD for this condition.

I think that after my TBI traumatic brain injury cannabis helped me recover. I told this to the neurosurgeon's head nurse but was dismissed without any consideration. This reminds me of the old saying "When all you have is a hammer everything looks like a nail."

It is important to consult a healthcare provider before using Charlotte's Web CBD or any other CBD product, as it may interact with other medications or have potential side effects. Additionally, the regulation and quality control of these products can vary, and it is important to use a reputable source.

In 1983 I was living in Vancouver in our studio called the Vancouver Videographers Club. Incidentally my videos and short documentaries are available on YouTube at @jerimiahcoffey400 or Jeremiah Coffey. We were using about our usual amount of high-grade hashish daily. The thing that was new is that two years earlier I had quit drinking alcohol completely after having been a heavy daily drinker for twenty years.

It was then that my mind must have been clearer that I began to question my behaviors and memory. I began to feel that something was not right. I did go for psychological testing and that was the time that I had the personal dilemma about knowing the answer to the question "Who wrote Faust?" because I had studied diagnostic testing not to cheat but simply out of curiosity.

By 1986 I was becoming alarmed that my memory was failing me. We decided to move back to Winnipeg. As soon as I got back home to Winnipeg, I remembered many situations that had happened in buildings as I passed by and I was very encouraged at my progress.

That is why I initially started university. It became a positive feedback loop where my memory improved. I had physical confirmation as I repeated scored near perfect examinations in every subject that I attempted. Barring some classes where staff recommended that I quit because they told me in confidence that senior professors were gunning for me. That is normal for me. I get warned that I am in danger by unknown 'others' fairly often. This can't be normal. It is not normal that somehow, I offend people unknowingly so badly. I never ask for clarification and try to give the informer the impression that I have confidence that I can handle any conflict that may arise with anyone, or any group as is often the situation.

I must admit that I thought that all claims that marijuana was medicinal were bogus attempts to get around the law. I never for a minute considered that the marijuana and hashish that I was smoking could have somehow had beneficial medicinal effects on me. Now I am not so sure. I think that it shrunk the adenoma of the pituitary that I had sparing me an operation. After a pattern of growing one millimeter per year before I started cannabis again to shrinking by two millimeters per year until it was not a concern.

I hurt my knee and was surprised to see how well pure CCBD oil rubbed into the skin around the knee managed the pain.

Oh yes pain. It must be a relative thing and apparently, I do not feel pain nearly as bad as other people do. One time in Vancouver I was getting two root canals on two adjacent bottom rear molars on my right side. I had heard that root canals were sometimes painful and was mentally prepared; and it did hurt quite a bit. This story is of course true. The dentist gasped in horror after the root canal when he looked down and saw that the tray with the freezing was unused.

I had a double root canal with no freezing and to me it was uncomfortable but ok. After that I would tell dentists not to give me freezing and take money off of the bill. A few would work on me without the needles but after a while they would insist. I think they thought that I was on heroin or some painkillers.

When I was in the hospital for my kidney stone removal, they gave me morphine but for a couple of months before that I had jackhammer type riveting pain in my kidney from the stents. I also felt pain from a shingles attack that hit my sciatic nerve that ran down my right leg.

In 2019 I began having some urgency regarding urinary urges. But like so many men I could not void well. I thought that my two or three short bursts were emptying me. I wound up nearly dead at the Seven Oaks Emergency ward and was admitted for a full week.

The doctors told me that they could not understand why pain had not brought me in sooner. They said it looked like the condition had developed over years and that maybe somehow, I got accustomed to the pain. My 400 to 600 -milliliter bladder was filled to over-capacity with at least 3.75 litres of urine. The pressure blew out my kidneys beyond repair and still I felt nothing out of the ordinary. My blood pressure was over 220 and my blood was saturated with things my kidneys should have filtered out. I had been staggering for two weeks before I went to the emergency room. I was drooling in my sleep and sweating profusely as my body tried to eliminate water.

I vividly recall the grade one teacher constantly forcing me to use my right hand and of course stop 'daydreaming' whatever that is.

The suppression of left-handedness or forcing a child to use their right hand as a dominant hand is not considered a direct cause of autism spectrum disorder. However, there is some evidence to suggest that a small percentage of individuals with ASD may also present with left-handedness or mixed handedness. However, this association is not well understood, and more research is needed to determine the exact relationship between handedness and ASD.

I have always been fascinated by right and left handedness. I am nearly ambidextrous in darts, pistol shooting, typing, and driving. My shooting instructors noted that whenever I was unsure or surprised in an IPSC scenario I would change hands to my left.

I tried learning darts for the first time to compare left and right scores. My left was better at darts. When I tried shooting pool, I found getting my body right for holding the cue stick was very confusing and uncomfortable. The big takeaway from the experiment which ended right there and then was that while the cue was in my left hand my mind said, "I can't use a cue with such a bad tip." That surprised me as I had never thought that before and I think that I thought differently because I was using my left hand.

Autism Spectrum Disorder (ASD) and Schizophrenia are two distinct mental health conditions that can have overlapping symptoms, but they have different causes, characteristics, and treatment approaches.

ASD is a neurodevelopmental disorder characterized by impairments in social interaction and communication, as well as repetitive behaviors and restricted interests. It is typically diagnosed in early childhood and is considered a life-long condition.

Schizophrenia, on the other hand, is a serious mental illness characterized by a disconnection from reality, known as psychosis. It typically develops in late adolescence or early adulthood and can cause a range of symptoms, including delusions, hallucinations, disordered thinking and behavior, and problems with motivation and emotion.

Treatment for these conditions also differs, with therapy and behavioral interventions being a key component of treatment for individuals with ASD, while individuals with schizophrenia often require medication and psychotherapy to manage their symptoms.

It is important to note that while there may be some similarities between the two conditions, each person with autism or schizophrenia experiences their condition differently, and it is essential to receive a proper diagnosis and individualized treatment plan.

It is possible for a person with narcissistic traits to also have Autism Spectrum Disorder (ASD), although it's not common for these two conditions to co-occur.

ASD is a neurodevelopmental disorder that affects a person's social communication and interaction skills, as well as their behavior and interests. People with ASD may have difficulty understanding social cues and norms, maintaining eye contact, and engaging in reciprocal conversations.

Narcissistic Personality Disorder (NPD) is a personality disorder characterized by a pattern of grandiosity, a lack of empathy, and a need for admiration. People with NPD often have an inflated sense of self-importance, a preoccupation with fantasies of power and success, and a sense of entitlement.

While some of the traits associated with NPD and ASD can overlap, they have distinct diagnostic criteria and can be differentiated through a clinical evaluation by a qualified mental health professional. Some people with ASD may struggle with social interactions and may appear self-centered, which can be mistaken for narcissism. Conversely, some people with NPD may struggle with social interactions because of their need for admiration and attention, but they don't typically show the repetitive behaviors and restricted interests associated with ASD.

Frontotemporal Dementia (FTD) is a progressive neurodegenerative disorder that primarily affects the frontal and temporal lobes of the brain, which are responsible for social cognition, decision-making, and language processing. The underlying causes of FTD are not fully understood, but the disease is characterized by the accumulation of abnormal proteins in the brain, which can lead to the death of brain cells and the loss of brain function over time.

Autism Spectrum Disorder on the other hand, is a neurodevelopmental disorder that is thought to be caused by a combination of genetic and environmental factors. ASD affects a person's social communication and interaction skills, as well as their behavior and interests. People with ASD may have difficulty understanding social cues and norms, maintaining eye contact, and engaging in reciprocal conversations.

In terms of symptoms, FTD can cause changes in behavior, personality, and language abilities. People with FTD may exhibit impulsive or socially inappropriate behaviors, difficulty with decision-making and problem-solving, and language difficulties. In contrast, people with ASD typically exhibit difficulties in social communication, including making eye contact, understanding social cues, and maintaining appropriate social boundaries. They may also display repetitive behaviors and restricted interests.

The age of onset is also different between the two conditions. FTD typically occurs in older adults, with an average age of onset between 50 and 60 years, while ASD is usually diagnosed in early childhood, although it can be diagnosed later in life.

Finally, treatment options differ between the two conditions. While there is no cure for FTD, medications can be used to manage symptoms, and behavioral interventions can help improve social and communication skills. In contrast, treatment for ASD usually involves a combination of behavioral therapies and medications, depending on the individual's specific symptoms and needs.

Behavioral therapies are a type of intervention that can be effective in improving social communication and interaction skills in individuals with Autism Spectrum Disorder . These therapies aim to teach individuals with ASD specific social and communication skills, as well as reduce problem behaviors that may interfere with daily functioning. There are several types of behavioral therapies that are commonly used for ASD, which I will describe in detail below:

1. Applied Behavior Analysis (ABA): ABA is a type of therapy that is based on the principles of behaviorism, which emphasizes the role of environmental factors in shaping behavior. ABA typically involves breaking down complex behaviors

into more manageable steps and using positive reinforcement to teach and reinforce those steps. ABA can be used to teach a wide range of skills, including language and communication, social interaction, and daily living skills. It is typically delivered one-on-one by a trained therapist and can be tailored to the individual needs and goals of the person with ASD.

2. Social Skills Training: Social skills training is a type of therapy that focuses specifically on teaching individuals with ASD the skills they need to interact and communicate with others effectively. Social skills training can be delivered in a group setting or one-on-one, and can cover a wide range of skills, including making eye contact, initiating and maintaining conversations, sharing and taking turns, and reading social cues.

3. Cognitive Behavioral Therapy: CBT is a type of therapy that is based on the idea that thoughts, feelings, and behaviors are interconnected, and that changing one can lead to changes in the others. CBT can be used to help individuals with ASD learn how to manage their emotions and behaviors, and to develop coping strategies for dealing with anxiety or other challenges. CBT can be delivered one-on-one or in a group setting.

4. Occupational Therapy: Occupational therapy can be helpful for individuals with ASD who have difficulty with daily living skills, such as dressing, grooming, and feeding themselves. Occupational therapy can also help individuals with ASD learn how

to cope with sensory sensitivities or challenges, such as difficulty tolerating certain textures or sounds.

5. Speech and Language Therapy: Speech and language therapy can be helpful for individuals with ASD who have difficulty with communication, including language development, articulation, and social communication. Speech and language therapists can work with individuals with ASD to develop communication strategies, such as the use of picture communication systems, and to improve social communication skills, such as turn-taking and initiating conversations.

Overall, behavioral therapies can be an effective way to improve social communication and interaction skills in individuals with ASD. The specific type of therapy used will depend on the individual needs and goals of the person with ASD, as well as the recommendations of a qualified healthcare professional. It's important to note that therapy for ASD should be individualized and tailored to the specific needs and goals of each person with ASD.

Chapter 13: Love and Understanding: Navigating Relationships with an ASD Partner or Loved One

Nowadays on the internet there is a lot of buzz about 'Narcissists'. The consensus is that the best thing to do with a narcissist is to avoid them. They often engage in controlling and stalking behaviours and can become violent.

The popular consensus that narcissists cannot have happy marriages is based on a few different factors.

Firstly, narcissists tend to have an excessive sense of self-importance and a lack of empathy for others. This can make it difficult for them to truly connect with and understand their partner's feelings and needs. They may prioritize their own needs and desires above their partner's, which can create a power imbalance in the relationship.

Secondly, narcissists often have a need for constant admiration and validation, which can lead them to seek attention and praise outside of their marriage. This can result in infidelity, emotional distance, and other behaviors that can strain the relationship.

Thirdly, narcissists may struggle with emotional intimacy, which can make it difficult for them to form a deep and meaningful connection with their partner. They may be more focused on the external trappings of the relationship, such as status and appearance, rather than the emotional bond between them.

Overall, these factors can make it challenging for narcissists to maintain a happy and fulfilling marriage. While it's possible for some narcissists to change their behavior and develop healthier relationships, it can be a difficult and ongoing process that requires a lot of self-reflection and personal growth.

Marriage can be challenging for individuals with ASD, and their difficulties in these areas can adversely affect their relationships with their spouses. Here are a few ways in which a man having ASD can impact his marriage:

1. Difficulty with social communication: Individuals with ASD may have difficulty with social communication, such as interpreting nonverbal cues, understanding social norms and etiquette, and recognizing emotions in others. This can lead to misunderstandings, misinterpretations, and communication breakdowns, which can cause frustration and conflict in the marriage.

2. Rigidity in behavior and routine: Many individuals with ASD find comfort in routine and predictability. They may have strict preferences around things like mealtimes, household chores, and daily schedules. This rigidity can clash with their spouse's more flexible approach, causing conflict and tension in the marriage.

3. Sensory processing issues: Many individuals with ASD have sensory processing issues, meaning

they may be over or under-sensitive to certain stimuli like noise, touch, or taste. This can make it difficult to navigate shared spaces like the home or bedroom. For example, a husband with ASD may need the lights off to sleep, while his wife prefers a dim light. This mismatch can cause problems in the marriage.

4. Difficulty with emotional regulation: Some individuals with ASD may struggle with emotional regulation, such as managing anger or frustration. This can result in outbursts, meltdowns, or shutdowns that can be difficult for their spouse to manage.

5. Lack of empathy: Some individuals with ASD may have difficulty with empathy or understanding and sharing their partner's emotions. This can make it challenging to support their spouse during times of stress or conflict, which can erode the intimacy and trust in the marriage.

It's important to note that every individual with ASD is unique and may experience different challenges in their marriage. However, with understanding, patience, and support from their spouse and potentially from a mental health professional, individuals with ASD can develop strategies and coping mechanisms to navigate their marriage and build a strong relationship with their partner.

My uncle Buck used to say, "Well, at least they did not spoil two families," whenever he saw an oddball couple out in public. While I don't completely agree with his sentiment, I do see the value in finding a partner who understands and can relate to the challenges of having a condition like ASD. In my own life, I have chosen to be with someone who has experienced their own difficulties - my partner is a Native Residential School Survivor who still deals with the residual effects of the abuse she suffered at the hands of nuns and priests during her time at those infamous institutions.

Despite our respective challenges, we make a great team. We each fill in the gaps where the other is weak, and we are able to forgive each other's blunders because we are familiar with the struggles of living with a condition. While we chose not to have children, we both feel that we would not have made the best parents. Instead, we focus on supporting each other and finding joy in our shared experiences.

One way my partner expresses herself is through her writing. She has written a book called 'Diesel Diaries,' which is a humorous self-study of America seen through the eyes of a long-haul semi-truck driver. Despite the challenges we face, we find joy in each other and the unique perspective we bring to the world.

As I reflect on the insights gained from this book, I am struck by the realization that my ASD is very likely a genetically inherited trait. This realization has allowed me to view my condition through a new lens and has helped me to understand the experiences of other members of my family like my late father who also exhibited symptoms of ASD.

With this newfound understanding of my condition, I am now better equipped to prepare for social situations and to anticipate how I may be perceived by others. While I have struggled with recognizing people's faces in the past, I have been able to make progress in recalling people's names, which has been a significant improvement for me. Additionally, I am more aware of how my behavior may be perceived by others, and I am learning to adapt my communication style accordingly.

Despite the challenges posed by my ASD, I have come to embrace my unique self and appreciate my differences. I do not wish to suddenly become "normal" and wonder how losing my ASD would impact my life. While it is possible that I may make new friends or perform better on the LSAT, I am not sure if I would want to lower my pain threshold, slow down my learning, or suddenly develop rhythm. I am comfortable living with ASD and believe that it has contributed to my strengths and abilities.

One of my strengths is being out in front of the crowd. As the joke says, "If you are one step ahead of the crowd, they will call you a leader. If you are two steps ahead of the crowd, they will call you a visionary. But if you are miles ahead of the crowd, they will call you crazy." I have found that my unique perspective and ability to think differently have allowed me to excel in areas where others may struggle.

In conclusion, this book has provided me with valuable insights into my condition, and I am grateful for the knowledge gained. I will continue to embrace my differences and strive to achieve my goals, utilizing my strengths and abilities to their fullest potential.

The End

www.ingramcontent.com/pod-product-compliance
Lightning Source LLC
Chambersburg PA
CBHW071403210526
45465CB00001B/231